CONTROLLED OR REDUCED SMOKING

Recent Titles in
Bibliographies and Indexes in Psychology

Psychosocial Research on American Indian and Alaska Native Youth: An Indexed Guide to Recent Dissertations
Spero M. Manson, Norman G. Dinges, Linda M. Grounds, and Carl A. Kallgren, compilers

Research on Suicide: A Bibliography
John L. McIntosh, compiler

Books for Early Childhood: A Developmental Perspective
Jean A. Pardeck and John T. Pardeck, compilers

Family Therapy: A Bibliography, 1937–1986
Bernard Lubin, Alice W. Lubin, Marion G. Whiteford, and Rodney V. Whitlock, compilers

States of Awareness: An Annotated Bibliography
John J. Miletich, compiler

Police, Firefighter, and Paramedic Stress: An Annotated Bibliography
John J. Miletich, compiler

Airline Safety: An Annotated Bibliography
John J. Miletich, compiler

The IQ Debate: A Selective Guide to the Literature
Stephen H. Aby, compiler, with the assistance of Martha J. McNamara

Research on Group Treatment Methods: A Selectively Annotated Bibliography
Bernard Lubin, C. Dwayne Wilson, Suzanne Petren, and Alicia Polk

Research on Professional Consultation and Consultation for Organizational Change: An Annotated Bibliography, 1974–1995
C. Dwayne Wilson and Bernard Lubin

CONTROLLED OR REDUCED SMOKING

An Annotated Bibliography

Compiled by
Pamela Rogers and Steve Baldwin

Bibliographies and Indexes in Psychology, Number 11

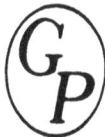

GREENWOOD PRESS
Westport, Connecticut • London

Library of Congress Cataloging-in-Publication Data

Rogers, Pamela, 1974–
    Controlled or reduced smoking : an annotated bibliography /
compiled by Pamela Rogers and Steve Baldwin.
        p.   cm.—(Bibliographies and indexes in psychology, ISSN
0742–681X ; no. 11)
    Includes indexes.
    ISBN 0–313–30988–4 (alk. paper)
    1. Tobacco habit Bibliography.   2. Smoking Bibliography.
I. Baldwin, Steve, 1957–   . II. Title. III. Series.
Z7882.R64 1999
[HV5735]
016.36229′6—dc21   99–22095

British Library Cataloguing in Publication Data is available.

Library of Congress Catalog Card Number: 99–22095
ISBN: 0–313–30988–4
ISSN: 0742–681X

First published in 1999

Greenwood Press, 88 Post Road West, Westport, CT 06881
An imprint of Greenwood Publishing Group, Inc.
www.greenwood.com

Printed in the United States of America

The paper used in this book complies with the
Permanent Paper Standard issued by the National
Information Standards Organization (Z39.48–1984).

10 9 8 7 6 5 4 3 2 1

CONTENTS

PREFACE

This annotated bibliography was compiled to provide a source reference for practitioners, field-workers and researchers. The aim has been to integrate a diverse literature from the fields of health education, health promotion, public health and applied psychology. The bibliography is intended to provide an up-to-date resource for academic, clinical and non-clinical workers, with a primary focus on 'what works' and outcome evaluations.

The authors would like to thank Amanda Kramer for her assistance.

INTRODUCTION

In the 2000s, smoking and tobacco use continues to be a major public health research arena. A series of "health scares" in the mid-1950s led to substantial research to establish a causal link between tobacco smoking and a wide range of health-related diseases/illnesses. The causal role of smoking in lung, mouth and throat cancer, chronic obstructive pulmonary disease (COPD), ischaemic heart disease and atherosclerosis was given particular attention. Low birth-weight and infant mortality (from smoking during pregnancy) was also widely investigated. Morbidity and mortality outcomes from tobacco smoking are well-established in the literature.

During the 1990s the focus of research was altered with a shift towards primary prevention and treatment. Since the establishment of the addictive nature of nicotine (and serious health consequences of cigarette smoking) there has been much data produced about smoking cessation. Studies have reported data on successful and unsuccessful cessation interventions. Other researchers have analyzed outcomes from unsuccessful subjects and reported reduction rates after high initial smoking levels. At follow-up, maintenance of both cessation and reduction rates have been reported.

Smokers who cannot (or will not) quit smoking have been neglected within smoking cessation campaigns. Chronic smokers with a long history of failed cessation attempts also have had few effective programs. A *risk reduction* approach (from attenuated, controlled or reduced smoking) may be of greatest benefit to this sub-population of smokers.

Controlled smoking is a term developed as a form of treatment for smokers who cannot (or do not wish to) quit. Controlled smoking is a modification of smoking behavior through alterations to the dimensions of *substance, rate, topography, location, motivation, or occasion.* Controlled smoking can be presented to smokers who cannot or do not wish to quit (despite, for example, smoking-related illnesses). The optimum goal may be a *harm reduction* strategy. There will be health benefits both for smoker and for any at-risk passive smokers. The most common form of controlled smoking is a reduction in rate of cigarettes smoked. Changing the cigarette brand influences nicotine levels, carbon monoxide and tar levels.

This monograph is an annotated bibliography of already-published studies about controlled, reduced or attenuated smoking. Studies aimed at smoking cessation have been included, if emphasis was also placed on smoking reduction for participants not achieving cessation.

The studies were arranged in seven categories:

1. Single Treatment studies, where the independent variable was a single treatment not easily broken into components. Some studies included a control group comparison.

2. Comparison of Single Treatment studies, in which two or more independent variables were compared in groups of randomly assigned subjects (equivalent subjects design). The independent variable was a single treatment as described above. Some studies included comparisons of multiple single treatments.

3. Multiple Treatment studies, where the independent variable was a treatment easily broken into different components, none of which was manipulated individually.

4. Characteristics and Process studies, where participants were selected for groups based on specified criteria for the independent variable. The same treatment or investigation was given to each group as the dependent variable.

5. Smoker x Treatment studies, where both the subject group and the treatment were independent variables. In studies of only one subject group, the population for the study was selected to fulfil specific criteria infrequently found in a random population.

6. Reviews, where no new studies were inspected, but a series of papers was presented. Most often a series of previously published studies was collated, with a discussion of results or theories.

7. Miscellaneous, in which studies that did not fit into any of the six categories were presented.

The databases (Psychlit, Sociofile, Medline, CINAHL, and CISDOC) were reviewed.

Chapter 8 gives an overall picture of the literature on controlled or reduced smoking. Attention is given to data collection, characteristics of smokers, and methods of treatment for the reduction of smoking. Limitations of current research and considerations for future research are discussed. In this chapter (and throughout the book unless otherwise instructed) articles are referenced according to entry number.

1

SINGLE TREATMENT

1.   Nolan, J. D. (1968). Self-control procedures in the modification of
      smoking behaviour. Journal of Consulting and Clinical Psychology,
      32(1), 92-93.

      Control of smoking behavior was attempted by manipulation of the
      relevant variables. One subject estimated smoking rate at 30 cigarettes
      per day (cpd) for several years. The subject could only smoke when
      seated in the designated "smoking chair" and monitored smoking
      behavior as well as time spent in the chair. Whilst in the chair others
      did not approach or speak to the subject, and the subject could not
      watch television, read, or participate in a conversation. The subject
      reduced smoking by approximately 50% of baseline for ten days from
      the establishment of the smoking chair. The chair was moved to the
      cellar to make it less readily accessible, and smoking decreased further
      to 5 cpd. One month after initiation of treatment the subject expressed
      disgust at her inability to quit. She quit successfully and maintained
      cessation for six months. The self-control procedure was designed to
      eliminate the control of some environmental stimuli, which act to
      maintain smoking behavior.   Successful reduction was achieved
      quickly and with only minor relapse. Cessation was not a goal of the
      program but may have been influenced by other reinforcers. It was
      suggested that cigarettes might be weak reinforcers, when compared to
      social and environmental factors.

2.   Resnick, J. H. (1968). Effects of stimulus satiation on the overlearned
      maladaptive response of cigarette smoking. Journal of Consulting and
      Clinical Psychology, 32, 501-505.

The effect of stimulus satiation was investigated to test the hypothesis that providing an excess amount of reinforcement could directly weaken smoking behavior. Sixty undergraduate volunteers (average age of 19.2 years) had smoked a mean of 22.25 cpd for 4.2 smoking years. Group 1 were told to triple their current smoking rate for 1 week; group 2 were told to double their smoking rate; group 3 served as a self-monitoring control group. Follow-up occurred two weeks and four months post-treatment. Similar reductions of no less than 50% baseline were reported at two weeks follow-up. All reductions were improved at four months follow-up. Nearly half the sample had quit by two weeks and most of these subjects had remained abstinent at four months follow-up. The control group did not significantly change from baseline at either of the follow-up interviews, although 25% of control subjects were abstinent at two weeks follow-up. The authors concluded that stimulus satiation of cigarette smoking is effective in controlling behavior. Results suggested that double satiation was as effective as triple satiation.

3.   Grimaldi, K. E., & Lichtenstein, E. (1969). Hot, smoky air as an aversive stimulus in the treatment of smoking. Behaviour Research and Therapy, 7, 275-282.

The study was designed to demonstrate the usefulness of hot, smoky air as an aversive treatment in the control and modification of smoking behavior using control groups. Another aim was to eliminate the large attrition rates observed in most pilot studies. Twenty-nine subjects (average age 43) reported a mean of 26 cpd during 24 years. Half the subjects had participated in a previous smoking control project and smoked 50% or more of their original baseline rate. Subjects were randomly assigned to treatment groups. Contingent punishment (CP) were given aversive smoke while smoking, and the smoky air was replaced by fresh air when each cigarette was extinguished. Non-contingent punishment (NCP) were given fresh air when smoking and hot smoky air when not smoking. The control (C) group received the same treatment as CP, except they had no aversive smoke.

All subjects attended seven sessions of ten trials (cigarettes) over three weeks and then attended a one-month follow-up. Subjects self-monitored cigarettes between sessions and rated the unpleasantness of each trial. Results indicated that reductions between baseline smoking level and the first inter-session interval were significant. Reductions between baseline smoking levels and end of treatment smoking scores were also significant. The difference between baseline and follow-up smoking was not significant. It was concluded that contingently administered smoky air in a punishment paradigm is not the causal factor in smoking reduction. Problems and limitations of this approach were discussed.

4.   McFall, R. M., & Hammen, C. L. (1971). Motivation, structure, and self-monitoring: Role of nonspecific factors in smoking reduction. Journal of Consulting and Clinical Psychology, 37(1), 80-86.

The authors reported four outcome patterns commonly overlooked in previous reviews of the smoking reduction literature. First, all smoking studies reviewed reported a reduction in smoking rate, which is not found in subjects not receiving treatment.   Second, studies have reported a V-shaped treatment curve of the amount reduction to baseline by time pre-treatment, post-treatment or follow-up.   Third, subjects achieve a reduction towards ten or fewer cigarettes per day but fail to achieve abstinence.   Last, data are often reported as "percentage of abstainers".   Subjects who achieved significant reductions were often not included. Exclusion of all data from treatment drop-outs enhanced the abstinence percentages of the research.

The authors report the outcome of 38 undergraduate students who were motivated to stop smoking and had smoked at least one pack a day for at least one year.   All subjects completed a smoking inventory and kept a continuous record of smoking behavior for 72 hours. Subjects also give a refundable $25 check.   The aim of the study was to dismantle a typical stop-smoking clinic program. The primary treatment variables assumed to be associated with smoking reduction were isolated and removed, resulting in a program containing only fundamental components (nonspecific factors). It was suggested that the use of primary treatment techniques would be questioned if the results of the treatment containing only nonspecific factors was the same as an unaltered stop-smoking clinic.

Four experimental groups were given identical treatments, except instructions for self-monitoring (SM).   Subjects were told to stop smoking 'cold turkey', and submit smoking record sheets twice weekly for three weeks. Cigarettes were purchased through the Smoking Clinic. Group meetings were minimal, brief and conducted by a 'low status' experimenter.   Follow-up questionnaires were conducted six weeks and six months post-treatment. The different methods of self-monitoring were minimal SM (given no special instructions about how to SM); negative SM (recorded on a wrist counter "occasions they were unable to resist smoking a cigarette"); positive SM (recorded on a wrist counter each occasion they successfully resisted smoking a cigarette); and fixed positive SM (subjects were required to record 20 positive SM points on a wrist counter each day). Results showed a marked reduction in smoking between the baseline period and the end of treatment, followed by a relapse to near baseline by six months. An analysis of variance found no effects due to groups. Subjects who achieved total abstinence post-treatment rated their motivation significantly stronger than subjects who failed to quit. It was concluded that subjects who received only nonspecific factors yielded outcome patterns comparable to more elaborate stop-smoking procedures. It was concluded that the results obtained in previous studies might be a function of their inclusion of non-specific factors rather than the elaborate treatment variable. Implications of this finding were discussed and directions for further studies were suggested.

5.   Levine, B. A. (1974). Effectiveness of contingent and non-contingent electric shock in reducing cigarette smoking. Psychological Reports, 34(1), 223-226.

The effectiveness of negative practice with both contingent and non-contingent electric shock was examined. Fifteen undergraduate subjects had a mean age of 22.1 years and mean period of smoking of 6.4 years. The electrical stimulation apparatus delivered an output of 110 volts ac and an approximate current of 50 milliamps via two metal EEG electrodes attached to opposite sides of the left wrist. Subjects self-monitored their smoking for two weeks, and were assigned to one of three groups. The control group (C) was placed on a waiting list for treatment. They were told to wait two weeks and self-monitor for another two weeks. The contingent-shock group (CS) were seen individually for four, 15-minute sessions over two weeks. Each subject smoked two cigarettes in succession, received one-second shock after inhalation and waited five beats on a metronome before the next inhalation. Each session involved 30 inhalations. The non-contingent shock group (NCS) received the same instructions and conditions as the CS group. The NCS group were delivered shocks only while the cigarette was in the ashtray between each inhalation.

Both CS and NCS groups self-monitored their smoking for one week post-treatment. Results showed CS subjects had reduced their mean smoking from 20.2 to 18.9 cpd. The C group increased from 16.9 to 18.3 cpd. Analysis of covariance indicated a significant experimental effect. The CS group was found to be significantly different from NCS and C groups, who did not significantly differ from each other. It was concluded that contingent shock holds promise as a reasonably quick method to produce *initial* change in smoking behavior but has not yet shown *long-term* behavior change.

6.   Rozensky, R. H. (1974). The effect of timing of self monitoring behaviour on reducing cigarette consumption. Journal of Behaviour Therapy and Experimental Psychiatry, 5 (3-4), 301-303.

The effect of post-monitoring (after cigarette consumption) and pre-monitoring (before cigarette consumption) was compared to eliminate smoking behavior. The subject was a female aged 49 who had smoked approximately 43 cpd for 25 years. Baseline data was obtained following a two-week estimate of daily cigarette consumption. In phase 1 the subject was allowed to quit on her own, again reporting an estimate of daily cigarette consumption. Phase 2 introduced post-monitoring where she was required to record the time and place after smoking a cigarette. Phase 3 replaced post-monitoring with pre-monitoring where she was required to record the time and place before smoking a cigarette. The results showed average daily consumption in Phase 1 similar to baseline; a small decrease in Phase 2; and a steady gradual reduction to abstinence in Phase 3. Follow-up at 50 weeks post-treatment revealed that she had maintained her abstinence. It was concluded that once the behavior had occurred, self-monitoring prior to the occurrence of the target behavior was more effective than self-monitoring after the behavior.

7.   Frederiksen, L. W., Epstein, L. H., & Kosevsky, B. P. (1975). Reliability and controlling effects of three procedures for self-monitoring smoking. Psychological Record, 25, 255-264.

The study was designed to examine the measurement reliability and controlling effects of 3 methods for the self-monitoring of smoking behavior. In experiment 1, 15 undergraduate students with a mean age of 18.67 years and mean smoking history of 22.68 cpd for 3.68 years, were randomly assigned to one of six conditions. The three types of recording methods were: continuous recording (CR) where the time was recorded at the commencement of each cigarette smoked, daily recording (DR) where the number of cigarettes smoked was recorded at the end of each day, and weekly recording (WR) where the average number of cigarettes smoked each day was reported at the end of the week. The measurement reliability was found to be higher for CR then either DR or WR. An analysis of the reported smoking rate by procedure did not reveal any significant differences. Questionnaires reported CR to be the most accurate, demanding, and most effective in controlling smoking behavior. DR was rated the best of the three self-monitoring procedures.

Experiment 2 was designed to evaluate the control of smoking over a five-week treatment period and a six-month follow-up. Thirty-six undergraduate students had a mean age of 19.20 years and a mean smoking history 23.31 cpd for 3.07 years. They were randomly assigned to groups as in Experiment 1 using CR, DR or WR. Three subjects from the CR group dropped out, reporting dissatisfaction with the demands of the procedure. CR resulted in the greatest smoking reduction compared to DR and WR although a significant difference was not reported until week 3. Significant differences were not reported at 6-month follow-up. This suggests self-monitoring did not automatically produce lasting changes in smoking behavior.

8.   Kopel, S. A. (1975). The effects of self-control, booster sessions and cognitive factors on the maintenance of smoking reduction. Dissertation Abstracts International, 35, 4184B-4183B.

The study investigated the use of a self-control procedure using rapid smoking and/or booster sessions in long term smoking reduction. The study also improved methodological weaknesses of previous studies. Hypotheses about cognitive factors, which influenced the maintenance of therapeutic behavior change, were also investigated. It was hypothesised that self-control procedures would produce greater maintenance of smoking reduction than experimenter-administered procedures; self-attribution of smoking reduction at termination would be positively associated with superior maintenance; and booster sessions of rapid smoking would improve maintenance. Fifty-three subjects were randomly assigned to self-concept rapid smoking (SC), external control rapid smoking (EC) or a minimal treatment control group (C). Baseline smoking levels were also measured. SC were trained at the first session to self administer the rapid smoking treatment at home for a total of 6 sessions. EC group were administered 6 rapid smoking treatment sessions at the clinic. C group was exposed to all components of the treatment package but smoked at the normal pace instead of rapid smoking. Booster condition subjects received 4 sessions identical to their treatment at 2-week intervals after termination. The groups averaged a 90% reduction of baseline smoking at termination. The rapid smoking treatment groups maintained reductions significantly more than the control group, but not significantly different from each other. Booster sessions did not affect maintenance and no relationship was found between maintenance and self-attribution or other cognitive variables.

9.   Ravensborg, M. R. (1976). Relaxation as therapy for addictive smoking. Psychological Reports, 39, 394.

A pilot study with a small number of subjects and no control group was presented, about the effects of relaxation for the treatment of addictive smoking. Forty-six subjects had a mean age of 43 years and a mean smoking history of 61.57 cpd for 24.86 smoking years. Subjects identified places on the human body where they often felt tension or cigarette cravings. Attention was focussed for relaxation methods on those spots. Mail and telephone follow-up was conducted at 4 months post-treatment; 4 subjects did not respond. Results showed the reduction in daily cigarette use (31.57 cpd to 22.86 cpd) was significant. It was also found that the people most able to relax their craving spots had the greatest success. Further research was recommended.

10.   Nesse, M., & Nelson, R. O. (1977). Variations of covert modeling on cigarette smoking. Cognitive Therapy and Research, 1(4), 343-354.

The study was designed to investigate the effectiveness of covert modeling as a technique to reduce smoking. Thirty-six undergraduate subjects who had smoked at least ten cpd for one year completed the treatment. Subjects were matched on baseline cigarette frequency, grade point average, and gender. Subjects were randomly allocated into four experimental groups and three experimenters (each experimenter treated one third of the subjects in each of the experimental groups). All subjects self-monitored their cigarette consumption, cigarette urges and "urge intensity" (on a 10-point scale). Self-monitoring accuracy was checked with two confederates selected by the subject.

The self-monitoring control group self-monitored for the duration of the study and met with experimenters for non-directive discussions in an equivalent number of sessions to the experimental groups. The Covert Modeling group received four sessions of covert modeling. Covert modeling comprised of imagining a scene which involved feeling an urge to smoke, and then making an alternate non-smoking response, which received a favourable consequence. The Covert modeling with high-value/high-rate self-reinforcement group (CM-HVHR) was asked to self-monitor previously selected high-value/high-rate activities, and to note whether they were able to engage immediately in the alternate non-smoking response, or if they was a temporal delay. The Covert modeling with low-value/low-rate (CM-LVLR) self-monitoring group did the same as the CM-HVHR but with previously selected low-value/low-rate activities.

Results show that covert modeling was not more effective than self-monitoring in decreasing smoking frequency, or urges to smoke. There were no significant differences in smoking frequency between the 4 treatment groups at any time during the study. A V-shaped curve in smoking rate over time was found for all 4 groups. Smoking frequency at the end of treatment was 40% of baseline, with relapse to 75% of baseline by 6-month follow-up. Due to the poor treatment effect of covert modeling, the motivational versus signalling aspects of overt self-reinforcement await further investigation.

11.   Kantorowitz, D. A., Walters, J., & Pezdek, K. (1978). Positive versus negative self-monitoring in the self-control of smoking. Journal of Consulting and Clinical Psychology, 46(5), 1148-1150.

A comparison of positive versus negative self-monitoring was assessed with a broad-spectrum behavioral self-control program for the reduction of cigarette smoking. Nine subjects with a mean age of 36.7 years were assigned to self-control with positive monitoring (P), self-control with negative monitoring (N), and a waiting list control group (C). Baseline smoking rates were 19.7, 26.8, and 15.6 cpd for P, N, and C groups respectively. Groups P and N attended eight 90-minute group meetings over 4 weeks. Both groups were instructed to: identify and avoid cues for smoking, use incompatible responses when feeling urges to smoke, use self-talk and imagery as tools for self-reward and punishment, and to complete contracts in their attempt to achieve abstinence by gradual reduction at their own rate. The N group recorded each time they yielded to an urge to smoke while the P group recorded each time they resisted an urge to smoke. Results show the C group decreased their rate by 1.1 cpd and one subject reached abstinence. The P and N groups reduced by 14.7 cpd (74.6% of baseline) and 16.8 cpd (62.8% of baseline) respectively; 4 subjects in P group and 2 in the N group reached abstinence. The follow-up rates of the P and N group remained 10.1 and 16.0 cpd below baseline. The results indicate no significant difference between positive and negative self-monitoring in the reduction of smoking behavior.

12.   Sutton, S. R., Feyerabend, C. Cole, P. V. & Russell, M. A. H. (1978). Adjustment of smokers to dilution of tobacco smoke by ventilated cigarette holders. Clinical Pharmacology and Therapeutics, 24, 395-405.

The study examined the extent of smoker compensation in the use of ventilated cigarette holders (to produce dilation of smoke). A standard analysis of a 1.3-mg nicotine cigarette (smoked by a machine) found nicotine reductions of 22.6% and 58.5% and CO reductions of 15% and 52.3% for holder 1 and 2 respectively. Eighteen subjects (sixteen males) had a mean age of 37.9 years and smoked an average of 29.6 cpd. Peak plasma nicotine and carboxyhaemoglobin levels were measured on each attendance day. No significant change in average cigarette consumption when using the holders was found. Subjects partially compensated by increasing the amount of smoke inhaled from each cigarette (indicated by increased plasma nicotine and carboxy-haemoglobin levels). Data reveals partial compensation on holder 2 but little or no compensation on holder 1. Individual variation in the amount of compensation was large; about half the subjects compensated on both holders. Amount of compensation was not significantly associated with usual cigarette consumption, nicotine level, baseline plasma nicotine or carboxyhaemoglobin level, withdrawal symptoms, or degree of satisfaction when using the holders. Compensation occurred only partially and with much individual variation. Plasma nicotine, carboxyhaemoglobin and tar intake to the lungs were presumed to decrease when the reduction in cigarette yields was approximately 50% or more.   It was concluded that insufficient evidence was found to confirm that compensatory smoking was driven by the need to regulate the intake of nicotine.

13.   Chambliss, C. & Murray, E. J. (1979). Cognitive procedures for smoking reduction: Symptom attribution versus efficacy attribution. Cognitive Therapy and Research, 3(1), 91-95.

The study evaluated two cognitive procedures to reduce smoking: symptom-attribution and efficacy-attribution. Symptom-attribution can be manipulated to incorrectly attribute internal changes to a neutral source, to alleviate various kinds of discomfort. Phase 1 involved placebo manipulations of 3 kinds, symptom-increase, symptom-decrease and symptom-irrelevant. The symptom-increase condition was hypothesised to be the most successful in reducing smoking, as subjects attributed withdrawal effects to the drug rather than reductions in smoking. Twenty-eight male and 18 female college students formed equal internal (9 or below) and external (11 or above) groups on the Rotter Locus of Control Scale. Within each group, subjects were randomly assigned to symptom-increase group (informed that the placebo would increase irritability, nervousness, and appetite), symptom-decrease group (informed the symptoms would decrease) and symptom-irrelevant group (informed nothing about symptoms).

Subjects self-monitored smoking behavior for 1-week baseline and the Tar Particle Matter (TPM) smoking score was recorded. During the experimental week, subjects were told to decrease their smoking behavior, were given a brightly coloured lactose capsule to take once a day; subjects continued to self-monitor. The results fail to support the misattribution or reverse placebo effect. Phase 2 involved efficacy-attributions, where attributing success to oneself increases a sense of self -efficacy, which enhances therapeutic progress. The subjects from phase 1 were asked to continue for one-week follow-up. Half the subjects from each group were given a debriefing about the placebo medication and told that 50% of all smoking reductions was achieved entirely by their own efforts. Self-monitoring continued for another week. The self-efficacy condition resulted in greater reductions than the drug-efficacy condition; this reduction for internal subjects was significant. The authors noted the importance of increasing self-efficacy in the reduction of smoking.

14.   Cornwell, J., Burrows, G. D., & McMurray, N. (1981). Comparison of single and multiple sessions of hypnosis in the treatment of smoking behaviour. Australian Journal of Clinical and Experimental Hypnosis, 9 (2), 61-76.

Problems associated with hypnosis studies were identified and discussed. Unresolved problems included: the use of techniques other than hypnosis during intervention, lack of control groups, hypno-tizability, measurement, and number of sessions required for treat-ment. The study investigated the relative effectiveness of single and multiple sessions of hypnosis against a no treatment control in the treatment of smoking. Thirty subjects with a mean age of 39.83 years and mean smoking history of 30.34 cpd for 21.9 years were referred by medical practitioners, or had volunteered for the study. Subjects were randomly assigned to one of three groups; multiple session group received four hypnotic sessions at weekly intervals, single session group, or a no- treatment control group. Follow-up occurred at one and two months post-treatment. Venous blood samples were taken at the initial interview and again at two month follow-up for analysis of plasma thiocyanate. Abstinence rates for the multiple session and single session groups were 70% and 40% respectively at one-month and 69% and 30% at two-month follow-up. One subject in the multiple session group achieved an 80% reduction in cigarette intake at 1 month. Two subjects maintained 80% reductions at two month follow-up. A 50% reduction at one-month follow-up by one subject in the single session group relapsed to 40% by two-months follow-up. No significant reductions were observed in the control group. Plasma thiocyanate tests were found to be a good objective measure to use with self-monitoring.

15. Lichstein, K. L., & Sallis, J. F. (1981). Covert sensitization for smoking: In search of efficacy. Addictive Behaviors, 6 (1), 83-91.

Six volunteer subjects were involved in a covert sensitization (CS) experiment for the treatment of smoking. All smoked at least 20 cpd, had a mean age of 33 years and had been smoking for an average of 16 years. Four procedures of CS were tested for efficacy. The first procedure was standard nausea aversion. The second used aversive themes but varied trial duration according to electrodermal arousal. The third procedure was the same as the second but an actual cigarette was used instead of a mental image. The fourth was the same as the third but with treatment sessions on five consecutive days rather than twice weekly. Disappointing results were reported with most reductions deteriorating to baseline by the two-month follow-up. The fourth procedure produced the most effective short-term reduction (80.5%) but care in interpretation of all results was required due to the small sample size. The authors discuss the advantages of each procedure and the need for further research.

16. Martin, J. E., Prue, D. M., Collins, F. L., & Thames, C. L. (1981). The effects of graduated filters on smoking exposure: Risk reduction or compensation? Addictive Behaviors, 6(2), 167-176.

Two experiments were presented which investigated the effect of graduated filters on cigarette smoking and health risk using the 'One Step at a Time' graduated filters and expired air carbon monoxide (CO) analysis. Experiment 1 involved one subject aged 29 years who had smoked 10-15 cpd for 13 years. CO levels were measured immediately before, and two minutes after smoking a preselected cigarette (of determined nicotine and tar level) either alone or with one of the four filters. The results obtained were consistent with the one-step filter manufacturer's claim of progressive reduction of CO gas intake. Mean CO boost across preselected cigarettes were reduced by 78% from the no-filter condition to filter #4 (highly aerated). Experiment 2 involved four smokers with heavy and long smoking histories. Subjects self-monitored cigarettes for three weeks then started with filter #1 and progressively changed filters every two weeks. Carbon monoxide levels were checked and smoking topography was analysed in Subjects 1 and 3. A decreasing trend in daily smoking rate was observed for three of the four subjects. All four subjects showing lower than baseline rates when on filter #4 . All 4 subjects showed large reductions in both tar and nicotine intake, as well as CO levels as they progressed through the different filters. No consistent changes in topography emerged indicating no compensatory changes. These studies have indicated success in reduction of tobacco exposure using the one-step-graduated filters; the filters reduced the effect on overall health risk.

17.   Prue, D. M., Krapfl, J. E., & Martin, J. E. (1981). Brand fading: The effects of gradual changes to low tar and nicotine cigarettes on smoking rate, carbon monoxide, and thiocyanate levels. Behaviour Therapy, 12 (3), 400-416.

An evaluation was completed of the use of low tar and low nicotine cigarette smoking prior to, and during, the gradual reduction of tar and nicotine consumption. The evaluation included carbon monoxide (CO), thiocyanate (SCN), and rate of consumption assessment. Nine outpatients from a Veterans Administration Medical Center participated, following a physician referral. Smokers had a mean age of 35.2 years, and mean smoking history of 28 cpd for 17.9 years. Smokers were asked to complete a series of progressive reductions in tar and nicotine using a brand fading reduction procedure. Carbon monoxide and SCN levels were assessed with feedback to the subject each week, and brand changes occurred every two weeks. Three subjects were assigned to Study 1 where CO and SCN were assessed three times a week. Study 2 involved six subjects. In Study 2, CO and SCN were assessed three times per week during baseline phase but only once a week during reduction phase.

In Study 1, comparison to baseline CO and SCN levels showed reductions, which stabilised during the final brand change for all three subjects. Generally, data for Study 2 replicated Study 1. All six smokers had lower levels of CO and SCN when smoking cigarettes with 3 mg or less of tar and 0.4 mg or less of nicotine. Overall the mean cigarette consumption for the nine smokers did not change from baseline to final brand change. The mean CO and SCN levels were 32.7 ppm and 31 mg%/ml at baseline and 17.8 ppm 17.7 mg%/ml during the final brand change indicating a 46% and 44% decrease respectively. At six-month follow-up, two were abstinent, and three had maintained reductions obtained at final brand change. Two smokers had relapsed but still smoked brands lower in tar and nicotine than baseline, and the remaining two could not be contacted. It was concluded that the reduction procedure has important implications for smoking treatment and decreased health risk.

18.   Burling, T. A., Stitzer, M. L., Bigelow, G. E., & Russ, N. W. (1982). Techniques used by smokers during contingency motivated smoking reduction. Addictive Behaviors, 7(4), 397-401.

The study investigated the smoking reduction strategies used by smokers who were reinforced for reductions of CO levels but given no specific reduction strategies or treatment. Twenty-four subjects averaged 26.0 cpd and had an average afternoon CO level of 28.1 ppm. Subjects smoked as usual for two weeks and baseline CO and daily smoking rates were recorded. For the next two weeks, half the subjects were offered monetary rewards for reductions in CO and the other half continued baseline monitoring. During the following two weeks all subjects were offered monetary rewards for reductions in CO level. The last two weeks involved self-monitoring and completion of a brief open-ended interview to describe techniques used to reduce CO levels. Results showed 67 techniques were used by the 24 subjects to reduce CO levels. These techniques were divided into 8 categories: changes in diet, engaged in activities where smoking was inconvenient, used gum or candy, limited time and situations of smoking, limited amount of each cigarette smoked, avoided smoking-related substances, some type of cognitive strategy, could not specify a plan. Diet changes and engaging in incompatible activities were the most successful methods of reducing CO levels. Finally, subjects who tried to reduce without a specific plan made the poorest reductions. This suggested that willpower also required a strategy to produce success in smoking cessation or reduction.

19.   Colletti, G., Supnick, J. A., & Rizzo, A. A. (1982). Long term follow-up (3-4 years) of treatment for smoking reduction. Addictive Behaviors, 7(4), 429-433.

The 3 and 4-year follow-up data from two smoking reduction clinics, which used a comprehensive, non-aversive behavioral treatment using stimulus control and self-control techniques, were presented. Subjects in both groups (clinics) attended five, one-hour sessions for four weeks which involved smoking reduction and maintenance strategies. An average of 90% of subjects was contacted across all the follow-up periods. Results of the four-year follow-up for group one and the three-year follow-up for group two indicated 23% and 28% abstinent and reductions of 57% and 53% of baseline smoking respectively. Many people in the sample (57%) were smoking 50% or less of their baseline rates at follow-up. It was suggested that for subjects not achieving abstinence post-treatment, a goal of controlled smoking might be appropriate.

20.   Sheehan, D. V., & Surman, O. S. (1982). Follow-up study of hypnotherapy for smoking. Journal of the American Society of Psychosomatic Dentistry and Medicine, 29 (1), 6-16.

The study reported the follow-up 18 months after hypnotherapy treatment to alter smoking behavior. Relapse rate over time, reduction of basal rate of smoking, complications of treatment, predictors of good response, and the relationship between subjectively perceived trance depth and outcome were assessed on 100 consecutive patients who sought hypnotherapy to stop smoking from two psychiatrists. The mean age of patients was 39.2 years and the mean smoking history was 31.9 cpd for 21.9 years. Ninety-four subjects were contacted at follow-up. Approximately 21% of subjects were still abstinent at follow-up; 30% failed to stop at any time post-treatment. Analysis of the relapse rate suggests that abstinence, which is maintained for three to four months, has a high probability of long-term success. Sixty percent of the non-abstainers had reduced their consumption to 40% of baseline. Fifty percent of subjects gained weight as a result of trying to stop smoking, with the mean weight gain of 10.7 pounds for long-term abstainers. The role of hypnosis as a therapeutic factor reported by subjects was minimal. It was concluded that hypnosis for the treatment of smoking was a brief, safe, therapeutic intervention that has some public health merit.

21.   Foxx, R. M., & Axelroth, E. (1983). Nicotine fading, self-monitoring and cigarette fading to produce cigarette abstinence or controlled smoking. Behaviour Research and Therapy, 21 (1), 17-27.

The goals of the study were to achieve a reasonable percentage of abstainers and reduce levels of nicotine and tar in non-abstainers. Twelve subjects met the criteria of smoking at least 15 cpd, of cigarettes containing at least 0.7 mg of nicotine. Subjects were given a nicotine fading and self-monitoring treatment, progressively changing cigarette brands to lower tar and nicotine, and plotted their daily intake of tar and nicotine for 3 weeks. Those subjects unable to quit at week 4 received a cigarette fading treatment where the number of cigarettes smoked was systematically reduced for 3 weeks. At 12-month follow-up, 33% of subjects had maintained abstinence; all non-abstainers smoked cigarettes lower in tar and nicotine than baseline. Half the non-abstainers had decreased their smoking rate. Mean reduction in daily nicotine intake was 81.6% from baseline and tar intake was 85.5% from baseline. Benefits were discussed for this non-aversive smoking reduction/cessation procedure for individuals with cardiovascular and respiratory problems, and a "least restrictive" treatment model for smoking.

22.   Glasgow, R. E., Klesges, R. C., & Vasey, M. W. (1983). Controlled smoking for chronic smokers: An extension and replication. Addictive Behaviors, 8(2), 143-150.

The main objectives of the study were to replicate a previous study on controlled smoking, enhance efficacy by using less abrupt reduction requirements and to provide feedback on behavior change rather than physiological change (CO levels). Eleven subjects recruited through public service announcements averaged 45 years of age and had a mean smoking history of 29 cpd for 26 years. The sample was categorized as fairly chronic cigarette smokers. Subjects attended seven sessions. In session one, subjects changed to a brand containing half the nicotine of their usual cigarettes. In sessions two and three, successive 25% reductions in percent of each cigarette smoked were established. In sessions four and five the number of cigarettes smoked per day were decreased by 25% successively. Session six involved subject goal-setting and strategy planning. Session seven gave information on relapse prevention.

Results showed that subjects achieved reductions in nicotine content, percent of each cigarette smoked and the number of cigarettes smoked per day. The data did not indicate compensation for reduction of one aspect of smoking behavior by an increase in the other two behaviors. With the exception of nicotine content, subjects rarely achieved the goal reductions of 50% but all subjects were able to make some reductions. The mean reductions were 28% for number of cigarettes smoked and 24% in the amount of each cigarette smoked. The changes were well maintained at 6-month follow-up. More gradual reduction goals and the inclusion of daily nicotine intake feedback did not produce the desired effects. The controlled smoking program was concluded to produce reliable and at least moderately successful long-term results.

23.   Goldberg, J., Zwibel, A., Safir, M. P., & Merbaum, M. (1983). Mediating factors in the modification of smoking behaviour. Journal of Behaviour Therapy and Experimental Psychiatry, 14(4), 325-330.

The study was designed to determine if covert sensitization would be more effective with subjects who responded strongly to an aversive film than subjects who reacted weakly. It was also aimed to determine if subjects who did not adapt to repeated aversive stimuli showed a greater decrease in smoking behavior than those who did adapt to the stimuli. Fifty-nine subjects responded to newspaper advertisements and then completed treatment and follow-up. The subjects had a mean age of 36.6 years and mean smoking history of 27.4 cpd for 10.7 years with a mean initiation age of 19.2 years. Fifty-three percent of subjects were professionals, 25.8% farmers (kibbutz members), 8.6% students, 8.6% housewives, and 3.6% factory workers. Each subject completed a background questionnaire, then individually viewed the stressor film (scenes from 'The Epileptic Seizure'). Two electrodes were placed on the index and middle fingers of the right hand. Subjects' responses to the film were placed in one of four groups; (1) high reactors, non-adaptive; (2) high reactors, adaptive; (3) low reactors non-adaptive; and (4) low reactors, adaptive.

Each subject attended 10 treatment sessions each lasting 1.5 hours over 3 weeks. Subjects sat in an individual cubicle and were played an audiotape, which included instructions for relaxation of muscles, five aversive presentations and five pleasurable presentations. Daily cigarette intake was obtained at three-, six-, and twelve-weeks post-treatment. An overall mean reduction of 61% in smoking behavior was reported. This reduction stabilized over time and was maintained for at least three months. An abstinence rate of 27% was reported post-treatment with 24% maintained at 3-month follow-up. Support was found for the first hypothesis; subjects who 'over-responded' to a visually presented stressor stimulus had greater success in reducing smoking behavior by an aversive control technique than those subjects who 'under responded'. The second hypothesis (non-adaptivity would be a significant factor in treatment effectiveness) was not supported.

24.   Ossip-Klein, D. J., Epstein, L. H., Winter, K., Stiller, R., Russell, P., & Dickson, B. (1983). Does switching to low tar/ nicotine/ carbon monoxide-yield cigarettes decrease alveolar carbon monoxide measures? A randomized controlled trial. Journal of Consulting and Clinical Psychology, 51 (2), 234-241.

A controlled clinical trial was presented of carbon monoxide (CO) changes in smokers who switched to low tar/nicotine/CO cigarettes with an assessment of altered smoking topography and rate. Forty subjects met the study criteria for: smoking history, health and desire to change. Subjects had a mean age of 38 years and had smoked an average of 37.5 cpd for 20.7 years. The cigarettes contained an average of 1.5 mg of nicotine and 17.1 mg of CO at baseline. Phase 1 supplied baseline figures of CO and smoking topography of the usual brand. Phase 2 initiated treatment. The Brand-Fading group (BF) received a five-week brand-fading program, and the Delayed Treatment group (DT) were asked not to change their smoking behavior until treatment began in seven weeks. During Phase 2 both groups followed their treatment instructions with an equivalent smoking rate. Phase 3 involved the post-treatment assessment of CO and smoking topography.

The study found that CO levels remained well above the low-risk levels even after switching to the lowest available tar/nicotine/CO cigarettes (90% from baseline). The smoking topography of the BF group did change; puff duration increased by one third and volume doubled, but the authors concluded that the data failed to explain the CO levels found. The authors suggested that a reduction in smoking rate might have produced a greater reduction in CO levels than equivalent smoking rates of a low nicotine/tar/CO cigarette. The authors concluded that CO levels in smokers was not a simple function of CO levels in cigarettes smoked.

25.   Marlott, J. M., Glasgow, R. E., O'Neill, K., & Klesges, R. C. (1984). Co-worker social support in a worksite smoking control program. Journal of Applied Behaviour Analysis, 17 (4), 485-495.

An examination was conducted of the effects of adding co-worker social support to a basic controlled smoking intervention trial. Twenty-four subjects with a mean age of 34 years and a mean estimated smoking history of 24 cpd of 0.75-mg nicotine for 16 years participated in the study. Fifty-four percent of subjects indicated intentions to quit while 46% indicated intentions to reduce but not quit. Subjects were assigned to controlled smoking (CS) or controlled smoking plus partner support (CS+PS) and both groups attempted to alter nicotine content, number of cigarettes and percentage of each cigarette smoked in a 25% reduction and then a 50% reduction from baseline. Subjects attended six weekly group meeting where the controlled smoking procedures were implemented and strategies discussed. CS+PS subjects were paired with a partner to discuss daily progress, aided by a Partners Controlled Smoking Manual. Feedback was provided via a monitoring book for support behaviors. The only significant result across conditions and time was nicotine content. This indicated that CS+PS maintained the reduction in nicotine content at 6-month follow-up better than CS group (who gave a larger initial post-treatment reduction). All subjects who quit smoking during treatment or follow-up (21%) remained abstinent at 6-month follow-up. Post-treatment reductions of 38% cpd and 49% CO levels were followed by relapse at follow-up. Implications of the results and directions for further research were discussed.

26.   Stitzer, M. L., & Bigelow, G. E. (1984). Contingent reinforcement for
         carbon monoxide reduction: Within-subject effects of pay amount.
         Journal of Applied Behaviour Analysis, 17 (4), 477-483.

         This study examined the relationship between pay amount and
         smoking reduction using five different payment schedules. Twenty-
         three female subjects averaged 31.6 years, with a mean smoking
         history of 23.7 cpd for 15.3 years, and all subjects had a CO level of
         above 18 ppm. Subjects were told that this was not a smoking cessa-
         tion program, but that optional changes might be encouraged. Sub-
         jects received free cigarettes (of their usual brand) during the study
         and a bonus $50 upon completion. Baseline data were obtained.
         Subjects were told that money could be earned each day depending on
         the carbon monoxide (CO) reading on their afternoon breath, which
         could be lowered by smoking reduction. CO readings of 6 ppm or
         lower gave the maximum payouts, while 7-21 ppm gave a variable
         payout in 5 categories, inversely related to the reading obtained. The
         payment schedule for Group 1 (n=12) changed daily while the Group 2
         (n=11) changed weekly. All subjects received advance notice of the
         next payment schedule. At each afternoon reading self-monitoring
         reports were collected and cigarettes were distributed for use until the
         next meeting. Contingent reinforcement promoted smoking reduction
         with the extent of reduction related to amount of payment available.
         As a function of pay amount, average CO levels decreased from 30
         ppm to 15 ppm, daytime cigarettes decreased from 12 to 5 per day and
         average minutes of abstinence prior to reading increased from 62 to
         319 minutes. It was concluded that interventions such as contingent
         reinforcement demonstrated that smokers may require the motivation
         to reduce or quit, rather than the knowledge or skills, which were
         apparently already present.

27.   Strecher, V. J., Becker, M. H., Kirscht, S. A. E., & Graham-Tomasi,
         R. P. (1985). Evaluation of a minimal-contact smoking cessation
         program in a health care setting. Patient Education and Counseling, 7
         (4), 395-407.

         A minimal contact smoking cessation program was offered to 213 in-
         patients and outpatients at a Veterans Administration Medical Center
         (VAMC). All patients, who smoked and were considered eligible and
         included, not just subjects motivated to quit, or who responded to an
         advertisement. Of the 119 eligible subjects, 20% refused the
         intervention; 72 patients (61%) accepted the program. Average
         smoking history of the subjects was 24 cpd for 34 years. Subjects were
         assigned by a three-month interval to either intervention or usual care.

Intervention was a minimal contact smoking cessation program designed for use in a health care setting. The program consisted of three components: consultation from a health care worker, a self-help smoking cessation manual, and an incentive to comply with the manual. Smoking status, health status, and demographic characteristics were obtained. Care varied according to the health practitioner and the health status of the subject. The daily smoking rate was significantly reduced for intervention subjects compared to control subjects. The smoking cessation rate for the intervention group (15.9%) was higher than the control group (8.9%) but not significant. Subjects characterized with a high level of functional impairment reported significantly higher reduction and cessation rates than the corresponding control group. The implications of this result were discussed.

28.   Baldwin, S., & Heather, N. (1986). Controlled smoking: Single case study with multicomponent intervention. Journal of Behaviour Therapy and Experimental Psychiatry, 17(4), 295-299.

A case study was presented of a multicomponent treatment package including topographical components and a health-related behavioral repertoire to produce controlled smoking. The subject was a 26 year old male who had a 10-year smoking history of between 0 and 45 cpd, smoking 20 cpd at the time of the study. He reported more than 50 quit attempts and 1 period of 6 months abstinence. He self-monitored the number of cigarettes smoked, hourly rate of smoking and number of puffs per cigarette to obtain baseline data. The package was designed to meet the individual needs of the subject. The subject agreed to a contract that forbid smoking from Saturday at midnight through to Friday at midnight. The 24-hour period outside of this time allowed unlimited smoking of his favourite brand. Environmental manipulations to avoid smoking-related cues and stimuli were recommended. Health-related behaviors (at least 15 minutes physical exercise per day) was initiated to compete with smoking behavior. The subject rewarded non-smoking by buying small luxury items with money saved and self-monitoring continued throughout the study period. Results show an 85% decrease in cigarette consumption maintained for the 30 month follow-up. An increase in time spent on daily exercise was reported during the follow-up period and a self-report of increased fitness and improved respiratory and cardio-vascular functioning was noted. The data supported the proposition that controlled smoking may be an acceptable goal for some long-term smokers who do not wish to abstain.

29. Benowitz, N. L., Jacob, P., Kozlowski, L. T., & Yu, L. (1986). Influence of smoking fewer cigarettes on exposure to tar, nicotine, and carbon monoxide. New England Journal of Medicine, 315, 1310-1313.

The study investigated the effects of cigarette reduction on tar, nicotine, carbon monoxide (CO), and smokers' satisfaction in a controlled environment. Thirteen subjects had a mean age of 37 years and mean smoking history of 39 cpd for 21 years and were paid for participation. The average smoking machine yields of subjects' usual brands were 17.3-mg tar, 1.1-mg nicotine and 14.9 mg CO. Subjects participated in four smoking blocks of three to four days each, smoking their own brand. The usual pace was adopted in the first block, followed by restricted smoking of 15, 10 or 5 of their usual brand for the other three blocks, the order balanced by Latin square. All cigarette butts, urine, and blood samples were collected. Concentrations of nicotine (AUCnic), carboxyhaemoglobin (AUCco), and mutagenicity of urine (UMA) were calculated. Results showed a decline in UMA and exposure to nicotine and CO as number of cigarettes reduced. Reductions however were proportionally less than changes in cigarette consumption. At 10 or 15 cpd (30-45% of baseline), blood nicotine concentrations were 60-70% of baseline and at 5 cpd (15% of baseline consumption) nicotine intake was reduced to 40% of baseline. The overall reduction in cigarette consumption resulted in only a 50% reduction in exposure to tar and CO. UMA, AUCco, and AUCnic analysis suggested that reduction in cigarette intake resulted in more frequent and intense puffing (compensatory smoking). It was concluded that a reduction in smoking did reduce exposure to toxins and related health risks. The reduction was not linear however and the magnitude of the benefit was less than expected.

30. Glasgow, R. E., Klesges, R. C., & O'Neill, H. K. (1986). Programming social support for smoking modification: An extension and replication. Addictive Behaviors, 11(4), 453-457.

The study was aimed to replicate and extend previous research on social support in a controlled smoking program. The previous study had found that co-worker social support did not enhance the effectiveness of the smoking control program. In the present study, significant others (who were not attempting to change their smoking behavior, outside of the work setting) provided social support. The frequency of negative social interactions with significant others was decreased, while the frequency of positive interactions was increased. Twenty-nine subjects averaged 33.5 years and estimated smoking an average of 25 cpd of 0.83 mg nicotine cigarettes for 15.5 years. Subjects participated in six weekly small group meetings and were randomly assigned to the basic program (BP) or basic program plus social support (BP+SS). Meetings were focussed on reducing nicotine content, followed by reductions in daily smoking rate, plus information provision and advice. BP+SS group included their partners in two meetings, which outlined the role of the partner and presented maintenance and relapse issues. The partners also received a partner support manual with outlined procedures. Smoking self-reports, butt analysis, CO, and saliva thiocyanate levels and responses to some smoking questionnaires were analysed.

Results showed 54% and 40% of BP and BP+SS respectively achieved abstinence post-treatment. Twenty-five percent and 23% maintained abstinence at 6-month follow-up. No differences between groups were found on any of the questionnaire or on biochemical measures. Subjects achieved a significant reduction in nicotine content of brand. They increased the number of cigarettes per day, however and also had increased saliva thiocyanate levels by follow-up. It was concluded that some aspects of social support were related to treatment outcome but overall improvement due to social support was not found.

31.   Belles, D., & Bradlyn, A. S. (1987). The use of the changing criterion design in achieving controlled smoking in a heavy smoker: A controlled case study. Journal of Behaviour Therapy and Experimental Psychiatry, 18(1), 77-82.

The study was designed to demonstrate the usefulness of an alternative changing criterion design to produce controlled smoking from a very high smoking frequency baseline. The subject was a 65 year old male with a 50 year smoking history of between 80-100 cpd. He self-monitored smoking for 7 days baseline and treatment was presented as a series of phases over 94 days. Each phase involved a stepwise change in criterion rate of smoking that shifted in direction (smoking more or less than the previous phase) for 3 to 8 days. If the target criterion was not reached, he sent a $25 penalty cheque to his least favourite charity. For each day the criterion was achieved he contributed $3 to a reward fund. Self-monitoring continued throughout the study. He reached his 19th criterion of 5 cpd on day 81, maintained at the 18 months follow-up. The changing criterion design was described as advantageous as it provided an alternative goal to abstinence, and was non-aversive. The design also minimized aversive withdrawal symptoms and therapist time.

32.   Rose, J. E., & Behm, F. (1987). Refined cigarette smoke as a method for reducing nicotine intake. Pharmacology, Biochemistry and Behaviour, 28 (2), 305-310.

A method of refining cigarette smoke was developed to supply smokers with a substitute to cigarettes that delivered most of the familiar sensory cues in smoke while greatly reducing the intake of nicotine and other smoke constituents. An innovative smoke condensate trap was developed. Cigarettes were smoked by a machine, which trapped particles in smoke in a vial while eliminating gases such as carbon monoxide (CO), formaldehyde, nitric oxide, ammonia and hydrogen cyanide, through a vacuum port by boiling the condensate. The condensate was then placed in a cigarette-sized tube and heated. The smoker could inhale vapors drawn from the condensate, which resembled smoke both visually and in flavour through a specially designed refined smoke device.

In Study 1 subject ratings of their own brand, low tar and nicotine cigarettes, and the refined smoke device were compared. Subjects were blind about which cigarette type they were smoking by use of an opaque screen and a mouthpiece. Ratings on scales of similarity, liking, strength, and harshness of refined smoke were significantly greater than ratings of low tar and nicotine cigarettes. Ratings of usual brands however were significantly higher than refined smoke on the same variables. Analysis found that in ten puffs, refined smoke delivered less than 0.05 mg of nicotine, 0.5 mg of tar and 0.5 mg of CO.

In Study 2, satisfaction with the relatively low nicotine delivery of the refined smoke device was assessed. Subjects were deprived of smoking overnight. The refined smoke was manipulated to appear stronger by reducing the size of the air intake vent and using a mixture of condensate and unburnt tobacco (75 mg + 50 mg respectively) to reduce clogging in the device. Refined smoke was rated as significantly more satisfying, harsher and stronger for strength (both of aroma of flavour and throat impact) compared to low tar and nicotine cigarettes. Breath CO showed virtually no change after five smoking periods with refined smoke but a 9-ppm increase after five low tar nicotine cigarettes. Analysis of the subjective and biochemical results suggested that refined smoke could provide an alternative to cigarette smoking, which minimizes the delivery of all harmful smoke constituents.

33.   Glasgow, R. E., Klesges, R. C., Klesges, L. M., & Somes, G. R. (1988). Variables associated with participation and outcome in a

worksite smoking control program. Journal of Consulting and Clinical
Psychology, 56(4), 617-620.

A work-site based smoking modification program was assessed to
determine variables associated with participation. Variables that
predicted immediate and long term success of abstinence or controlled
smoking were assessed. From a total of 154 smokers who completed a
baseline questionnaire, 93% decided to participate. Fourteen other
subjects who did not complete the initial questionnaire also received
treatment.   Subjects had smoked for an average of 14 years and
participated in six weekly small group meetings which lasted about 50
minutes, conducted during work hours. Initial meetings focussed on
brand changes to lowered tar/nicotine content and reduced number of
cigarettes smoked. Subjects set a goal of abstinence or reduced smoking and were provided with cognitive and behavioral coping strategies,
maintenance, and relapse prevention.   Prizes were awarded to the
work-site with the highest participation rate, greatest post-treatment
reductions in CO, and the highest cessation rate over six months. The
prizes were designed to benefit both smokers and non-smokers.
Results show that 32% of subjects were abstinent post-treatment.
These subjects were found to be significantly younger and had lower
scores on the strength of habit scale than non-abstainers. Overall, a
mean reduction of 50% in post-test CO levels was found for non-
abstainers, maintained at 6-month follow up. The directions of the
relationship between the predictor variables and the sample were
discussed.

34.   Hill, D., Weiss, D. J., Walker, D. L., & Jolley, D. (1988). Long term
        evaluation of controlled smoking as a treatment outcome. British
        Journal of Addiction, 83, 203-207.

One thousand three hundred and twenty-six subjects with a mean age
of 38.7 years, had smoked an average of 28 cpd completed a smoking
cessation course called "Fresh Start". Eight two-hour sessions were
held over four weeks and addressed cognitive principles to provide
information and to devise strategies for abstinence.   At one-year
follow-up, 62% were abstinent and 18% smoked between one and nine
cpd. They were considered controlled smokers. Controlled smokers
did not achieve the lowest percentage reduction in the long-term. The
percentage of long-term abstainers among the controlled smokers (5%)
was no higher then any other group. Smokers did not use controlled
smoking as a stepping stone towards abstinence.   The authors
comment that "abstinence rather than control" was emphasized as the
long-term goal of the treatment. The results were consistent with

other reports that post-treatment non-abstainers typically relapsed during the follow-up period. The authors concluded that damage done by tobacco was directly linked to the amount consumed. There was no safe threshold from smoking, suggesting that controlled smoking was not an appropriate treatment.

35.   Gawin, F., Compton, M., & Byck, R. (1989). Buspirone reduces smoking. Archives of general Psychiatry, 46 (3), 288-289.

The use of buspirone, a nonsedative antianxiety agent, for the modification of smoking behavior was described. Seven subjects completed the study. They all had smoked over 1.5 packs of cpd for over five years had previous unsuccessful quit attempts and met the DSM-III-R criteria for an anxiety disorder. Subjects were given buspirone in doses starting at 15 to 30 mg/d increased to 10 mg increments over the six week treatment period to a maximum of 60 mg/d. Subjects self-monitored smoking behavior and rated their smoking desire or craving for the previous day. All subjects reported sustained reductions (but not elimination) of the urge to smoke. All subjects decreased smoking to seven or less cpd for at least one week. It was reported that buspirone seemed to minimize craving and withdrawal anxiety, fatigue and weight gain in subjects who reduced or quit smoking.

36.   O'Conner, K., & Physant-Skov, M. (1989). Smoking reduction based on a situational model of craving. Psychological Reports, 65(3), 963-966.

The report described the effect of a situational approach to smoking reduction in a local health setting. The program identified five key smoking situations: Boredom, Relaxation, Emotional stress, Attentional stress, and Keeping company (BREAK). A substitute action for the smoker was devised for each situation. Subjects self-monitored for two weeks baseline, followed by six weeks treatment. Follow-up occurred at two-, six-, and twelve-months. Six subjects with a mean age of 39.2 years completed a battery of questionnaires and began treatment. The first two weeks of treatment targeted awareness training, followed by two weeks of behavioral substitutions and a program of controlled reductions followed by relapse prevention information. At the end of treatment, three smokers had quit completely, two had made substantial reductions and one made only a slight reduction. Of the abstainers at twelve-month follow-up, one remained abstinent, one smoked the occasional cigar and the other smoked three cpd. The three reducers maintained their low levels of smoking, still significantly different from baseline. It was concluded that smokers to maintain smoking reductions could achieve selective control over situational cues.

37.   Spanos, N. P., Sims, A., deFaye, B., Mondoux, T. J., & Gabora, N. J. (1992). A comparison of hypnotic and nonhypnotic treatments for smoking. Imagination, Cognition and Personality, 12 (1), 23-43.

Three experiments using hypnotic and non-hypnotic treatments for smoking cessation were presented. Experiment 1 involved 84 volunteer subjects from a university setting with a mean age of 23 years. They had smoked for an average of 7 years. There were five groups: Passively worded hypnotic induction (G1), Passively worded treatment with no hypnotic induction (G2), Actively worded hypnotic induction (G3), Actively worded treatment with no hypnotic induction (G4), and a control group who received no hypnotic induction or treatment (C). Dropout rate was large; only 65.5% of subjects completed treatment and follow-up. Subjects reported significant reductions in smoking across sessions but no differences were found between the five groups. There was no evidence that manipulation of hypnotherapy or the tone of treatment produced more effective smoking cessation.

Experiment 2 involved 55 subjects in the comparison of single or multi (four) sessions under hypnotic and non-hypnotic procedures in the treatment of smoking. A no-treatment control group was used. Initial smoking reductions for the treatment groups compared to the control group were not maintained at an eight-week follow-up. The abstinence rates reported were substantially lower than other published findings. Experiment 3 used the one session version of Experiment 2 on a non-university population. Thirty-nine subjects aged between 19 and 58 years completed treatment. Reductions in smoking were equivalent to Experiment 2 at initial follow-up (four weeks). It was concluded that use of non-student subjects had little effect on treatment results. There was a substantial influence in response to the control conditions, where student subjects show a reduction from baseline. All experiments reported very low abstinence rates compared to other studies.

38.   O'Conner, K., & Langlois, R. (1993). Situational typing and graded smoking reduction. Psychological Reports, 72(3), 747-751.

It was hypothesized that subjects showing a preference to smoke when actively involved in a task would benefit more from a smoking program, which emphasized coping with task demands, rather than subjects with little active preference. Out of 27 respondents to a basic smoking questionnaire, 14 subjects were selected to be in the active group and 13 in the inactive group. Subjects reported a mean of 16 smoking years and averaged 39.5 years. Both groups attended 10 weekly 90-minute sessions, which involved awareness exercises, gradual reduction of smoking in low-risk, medium-risk, and high-risk situations successively, relapse prevention and coping strategies. Subjects completed questionnaires and self-monitored smoking throughout the treatment, and 2 and 6 month follow-up. Results indicated that active smokers showed initial high craving to smoke and low efficacy to not smoke during task activities. Inactive smokers showed the same pattern during boredom. The situational differences had disappeared by week 5. No differences in situational craving were found at 2-month follow-up. Both groups showed a significant decrease in craving over all sessions and situations. Both groups showed a linear decrease in number of cigarettes smoked over sessions. There were no significant differences between groups at post-treatment or 2-month follow-up. Varying relapse occurred by 6 months follow-up. It was concluded that the consistent long term efficacy and mood changes achieved were due to the coping strategies involved in maintenance.

39.   Brigham, J., Gross, J., Stitzer, M. L., & Felch, L. J. (1994). Effects of a restricted work-site smoking policy on employees who smoke. American Journal of Public Health, 84, 773-778.

The biological, subjective and behavioral impact of a smoking policy restriction on individual smokers was compared to a control group of smokers whose work-site smoking policy remained unrestricted. The treatment group consisted of 34 smokers with a mean age of 38 years and a mean smoking history of 22 cpd for 19 years. The control group consisted of 33 smokers with a mean age of 37 years and mean smoking history of 27 cpd for 18 years. Experimental subjects attended a laboratory data collection session once per week for four weeks before and four weeks after implementation of a work-site ban. Control subjects attended data collection sessions at their work-site for eight consecutive weeks. Data collected included self-monitoring reports, butt collection, saliva samples for nicotine and cotinine, breath carbon monoxide (CO), withdrawal symptom questionnaire, Profile of Mood States, and a work attitude and performance questionnaire.

Based on self-reports, consumption of cigarettes during work hours dropped significantly as a function of the ban in the experimental group, from smoking 7.57 cigarettes during work to 3.64 cigarettes after the ban. The smoking rate for the control group did not differ over time. Restricted subjects reported an average of 5.89 cigarettes during work at their workstation before the ban, compared with 0.69 after the ban, with the reverse pattern observed for smoking behavior outside the building. Significant interactions on both saliva nicotine and breath CO levels were observed. Changes were noted in work-shift smoking behavior. No change was observed for the control group. Smokers did not compensate for the reduction in smoking during work hours by increasing smoking outside of work or by more intensive smoking. Cotinine analysis suggests that the smoking ban intervention provided limited immediate health benefits to smokers from reductions to tobacco exposure, while producing minor withdrawal discomfort.

40.   Capafons, A., & Amigo, S. (1995). Emotional self-regulation therapy for smoking reduction: Description and initial empirical data. International Journal of Clinical and Experimental Hypnosis, 43 (1), 7-19.

Self-regulation therapy, based on a cognitive skill-training program that increased hypnotizability, can be used to treat many problems. Emotional and physiological self-regulation therapies consisted of three phases. In phase 1 the subject formed an association between sensations and images, words or cues that can later be reproduced without needing the physical stimulus. In phase 2 the subject reproduced the sensations without the real stimulus to many images, thoughts or cues until direct suggestion alone produced automatic reproduction of the sensation. Phase 3 (also called the generalization phase) established a post-self-regulation-therapy cue so that the sensation could be experienced prior to the presentation of therapeutic suggestion. Physiological self-regulation therapy was used to create a 'medical' context that will be more credible to patients resistant to psychological determinants of their problem. Self-regulation therapy elicited positive mood and heightened arousal, which increased self-efficacy expectancies.

It was reported that subjects who received emotional self-regulation therapy as a treatment for smoking gave up smoking at a very high rate (47%), similar to the best reported hypnotic interventions, with a very low dropout rate. Subjects who received physiological self-regulation therapy produced an abstinence rate of 60%. Twenty-six percent partially reduced consumption and 14% became self-controlled smokers. At three-month follow-up 45% of abstainers had relapsed; 88% of reducers had relapsed but no relapse was observed for the self-controlled smokers. As individual goals are set for treatment, this procedure could be used to treat smokers who did not wish to quit, but become controlled smokers. Withdrawal symptoms were practically absent in subjects during therapy and were reported in low rates during follow-up. It was concluded that self-regulation therapy could be used successfully to treat smoking.

41.   Prince, F. (1995). The relative effectiveness of a peer-led and adult-led smoking intervention program. Adolescence, 30(117), 187-194.

The effectiveness of a peer-led smoking intervention program (compared with the same program led by adults) was assessed for use with high-school age smokers. Ninety-three students in year 11 or 12, were divided into three groups: Peer-led (P), Adult-led (A), and Control (C). Peer and adult leaders attended two days training in group leadership and program content. All participants completed the Tobacco Use Survey, and the Tobacco Experience Survey pretest, and the Program Participant's Feedback Form and the Smoking Self-Efficacy Questionnaire was completed post-test (at the end of the six session program), and at one month follow-up. Pre-test smoking rate was between 11-13 cpd, by posttest, 17% of all participants had quit, and by one-month follow-up, 18.1% had quit. The participants in the peer-led program were not found to reduce smoking significantly more than the adult-led group. Both groups however did show significant reductions in cpd from pretest to posttest, maintained at follow-up compared to the control group. The peer-led and adult-led interventions were equally effective.

42.   Tilashalski, K., Lozano, K., & Rodu, B. (1995). Modified tobacco use as a risk-reduction strategy. Journal of Psychoactive Drugs, 27(2), 173-175.

The use of smokeless tobacco as a risk reduction strategy to cigarette smoking was presented. Oral cancer is the only serious health risk from smokeless tobacco (ST), with negligible cardiovascular risk. Cancer from ST represented only 5% of all smoking-related cancers, less than 10% of smoking- related lung cancers and only half of the oral cancers attributed to smoking. ST would decrease annual deaths from smoking and health costs. Twenty-two adult ST users who were former smokers were analyzed to explore their motivation and transition to ST. Demographic information, smoking history, motivational influence (in three categories, perceived health risk, adverse health experiences or social pressure), and ST history (including type-chewing tobacco, moist snuff, or plug tobacco, amount, and duration) were collected in telephone interviews. The authors pointed out that due to the small sample size, the group was not statistically representative of the population of smokers who changed to ST. It was found that transition to ST use often occurred, even after a long smoking history and when ST use had been maintained for an average of over 9 years. The authors suggested that for smokers unwilling or unable to abstain from tobacco, modification to a less harmful nicotine delivery system, like ST, was appropriate. Unlike nicotine gum or patches, ST provided substantial amounts of available nicotine with plasma nicotine levels comparable to smokers, and delayed withdrawal effects due to sustained mucosal absorption after removal of ST.

2

COMPARISON OF SINGLE TREATMENTS

43. Sachs, L. B., Bean, H., & Morrow, J. E. (1970). Comparison of smoking treatments. Behavior Therapy, 1, 465-472.

Three treatments, covert sensitization (CS), self-control (SC), and placebo attention (PA), were compared for their effect on smoking behavior. Thirty-seven subjects from a student population with an average age near 20 years completed one week of self-monitoring and were randomly assigned to one of three groups. Each subject attended three weekly treatment sessions, and was instructed to continue the procedure alone. They were contacted by phone one-month post-treatment for follow-up. PA group continued to carefully record their smoking behavior. They were given verbal approval for completed self-monitoring forms or statements showing increased awareness of their smoking patterns. SC group categorised smoking behavior according to the discriminative stimuli leading to smoking. Subjects were told to stop smoking in the presence of each situation in progressive order of perceived difficulty. Subjects could still smoke when they wished but only when removed from target situations. CS group ranked reinforcing stimuli in order of reinforcement strength. Subjects then paired the pleasurable sensations of reinforcing stimuli with visualizations of aversive scenes.

Twenty-four subjects completed treatment. Results showed that cigarette consumption was significantly less for each week of treatment and during follow-up than during baseline. Post-treatment was significantly less than baseline and post-treatment was also significantly less than follow-up. The SC and CS group means were significantly less than baseline while PA was not. It was concluded that subjects significantly altered their smoking behavior with CS or SC treatment but PA treatment was ineffective. Limitations due to the light smoking patterns of subjects in the study were discussed.

44.   Lichtenstein, E., Harris, D. E., Birchler, G. R., Wahl, J. M., & Schmahl, D. P. (1973). Comparison of rapid smoking, warm smoky air, and attention placebo in the modification of smoking behavior. Journal of Consulting and Clinical Psychology, 40, 92-98.

The study was designed to evaluate individual or combined contributions of warm smoky air and rapid smoking and experimenter effects in the modification of smoking behavior. Forty subjects had a mean age of 32.3 years and mean smoking history of 26.9 cpd for 14.7 years. Subjects were randomly assigned to one of four groups and three experimenters (E's). Group 1 received warm smoky air plus rapid smoking, Group 2 received warm smoky air only, Group 3 received rapid smoking only. Group 4 received an attention-placebo control group, which received no aversive stimulation. All except one subject was abstinent post-treatment, and follow-up data were obtained for 39 subjects. The three aversion groups performed similarly during the follow-up period with a gradual relapse in the first three-months followed by maintained reductions of near 25% of baseline. Group 4 showed greater relapse at follow-up; they smoked at baseline levels by 6 months post-treatment. Twelve subjects in the aversion groups were non-abstinent at six-month follow-up, ten of which had relapsed to baseline smoking levels. No experimenter effects were found. A significant difference in mean smoking rate between the control group and the aversive groups demonstrate that aversion is a significant factor in the modification of smoking behavior. The similar outcome for the three aversion groups indicates treatments are virtually interchangeable. The discussion was focused on smoking cessation rather than smoking reduction. A comparison of results with a previous study and recommendations for future research were also included.

45.   Russell, M. A. H., Wilson, C., Patel, U. A., Cole, P. V., & Feyerbend, C. (1973). Comparison of effect on tobacco consumption and carbon monoxide absorption of changing to high and low nicotine cigarettes. British Medical Journal, 4, 512-516.

The study compared the effect of tobacco consumption and carbon monoxide (CO) absorption levels in smokers who changed to high and low nicotine cigarettes. Ten regular cigarette smokers volunteered to take part in the study over four, five-hour periods on two consecutive days for two weeks. On the first day the subject smoked their usual brand. On the second day they smoked either the high or low nicotine brand, with the other brand (high or low nicotine) smoked in the second week. Subjects were supplied with the appropriate cigarettes and saved all butts for weight analysis (and as a check on the number of cigarettes smoked). Blood samples were collected before and after each session for carboxyhaemoglobin (COHb) analysis. Satisfaction, strength and taste evaluations were also collected.

Results showed that changing to low nicotine cigarettes produced a slight increase in the number of cigarettes smoked but the difference was not significant. On changing to high nicotine cigarettes the 38% decrease in the number of cigarettes smoked was significant. Weight analysis of butts showed a tendency to smoke slightly more of the low nicotine cigarettes which was not significant, and significantly less of the high nicotine cigarettes. The difference in COHb indicated a decrease when smoking high or low nicotine cigarettes compared to usual brand, but the decrease was not significant. The subjects rated the low nicotine cigarettes as too weak, not satisfying or good tasting while the high nicotine cigarettes were regarded satisfying and good tasting although too strong. It was concluded that regular smokers who inhaled, modified their smoking behavior to regulate their nicotine intake. COHb levels decreased with high nicotine cigarettes due to the decreased rate of smoking. COHb levels also decreased with low nicotine cigarettes due to the low CO yield of the cigarettes.

46.   Sipich, J. F., Russell, R. K., & Tobias, L. L. (1974). A comparison of covert sensitization and "nonspecific" treatment in the modification of cigarette smoking. Journal of Behavior Therapy and Experimental Psychiatry, 5(2), 201-203.

The effectiveness of covert sensitization in the reduction of smoking behavior was assessed. The effects of nonspecific elements like placebo and suggestion in the reduction of smoking behavior was also assessed. Forty-nine subjects averaged between 27 and 31 cpd and completed treatment in one of five groups. The Covert Sensitization (CS) group self-monitored for one week to establish baseline data, followed by two weeks (six sessions) of treatment. This treatment involved progressive muscle relaxation training and vivid visualization of aversive feelings like nausea and vomiting when smoking. The Attention Placebo (AP) group self-monitored for one week followed by two weeks of treatment in which subjects were told that smoking was a habit not under their control. They were instructed that by viewing subliminal messages on a tachistoscope they would be subconsciously reconditioned (the messages used were combinations of nonsense syllables). Self Control suggestion (SC) group self-monitored for one week and were then told to quit smoking using their own efforts, as tricks and gimmicks could not help them. Subjects were contacted five times by telephone where praise for the success of their self-help methods was given. Monitoring control (MC) group self-monitored only. After one week of self-monitoring they were told that treatment was delayed but to continue self-monitoring. No contact control (NC) group received no treatment or contact except collection of pre- and post-treatment data.

Following treatment, CS, AP and SC were contacted weekly for ten follow-up weeks and again at six months. Results indicated that CS, AP and SC differed significantly from controls MC and NC, but not from each other at the end of the treatment period. No significant differences were found between treatment groups during ten week or six month follow-up. Although smoking reductions were not maintained, the rate of smoking at six months was still significantly less than baseline. It was concluded that non-specific effects of attention or suggestion were valid interpretations for the effectiveness of covert sensitization.

47.   Wisocki, P. A., & Rooney, E. J. (1974). A comparison of thought stopping and covert sensitization techniques in the treatment of smoking: A brief report. The Psychological Record, 24(2), 191-192.

The study compared the effectiveness of thought-stopping to covert sensitization in the reduction of smoking behavior. Eleven subjects, who met the programs' time schedule were randomly assigned to one of three treatment groups: thought stopping (TS), covert sensitization (CS) and attention placebo (AP). Seventeen subjects were placed in a no contact control group. Subjects were recruited from notices in a student newspaper. They smoked a mean of 24 cpd for 10 smoking years. Subjects attended ten, 20-minute sessions over five weeks. TS were instructed to shout "stop" to themselves at imagined scenes involving environmental stimuli for smoking. CS were told to make a specific unpleasant association to smoking, like vomiting, to the same scenes as TS, and AP were told to relax. Subjects were told to practice the procedure at home, when they were tempted to smoke. Results indicate significant smoking reductions post-treatment for TS and CS groups but not for the AP group. Results from a four-month follow-up show no statistically significant reductions for any group. Although the small size of treatment groups was acknowledged, the authors discussed the benefits of the thought-stopping procedure.

48.   Sutherland, A., Amit, Z., Golden, M., & Roseberger, Z. (1975). Comparison of three behavioral techniques in the modification of smoking behavior. Journal of Consulting and Clinical Psychology, 43 (4), 443-447.

A comparison of three behavioral techniques (relaxation, satiation, and its combination) was performed to determine relative effectiveness in reduced cigarette smoking. Fifty-three subjects were randomly assigned to the four groups matched on age and sex. A fifth group of smokers with no desire to change their smoking behavior served as a control group. No significant difference in average daily consumption or number of years smoking was observed between groups. Group 1 received relaxation treatment only. Group 2 received satiation only, where subjects were told to inhale deeply every 4 seconds for the duration of one cigarette, and to repeat the procedure after a 15 minute break. This procedure was described as a method to change the short-term reinforcement consequences of smoking from positive to negative for smoking behavior. Group 3 received both relaxation training and satiation treatment. Group 4 was instructed to self-monitor smoking and reports it weekly to an experimenter by phone. This group was designed as a control for the effect of simple record-keeping by moti-vated subjects. Group 5 also received no treatment except self-monitoring. It was designed as a control for the effects of simple record keeping by unmotivated subjects.

Cigarette consumption was reduced by 57.42% for Group 1, 68.99% by Group 2, and 15.57% by Group 3 with no change reported in the two control groups. By the three-month follow-up, relapse had occurred to 65.04% in Group 1. Group 2 relapsed to 102.43% at three-month follow-up (follow-up smoking rate exceeded baseline smoking rate!). Group 3 was the only group to maintain a significant reduction in smoking behavior over the follow-up period. The consistent data of the control groups showed that the treatment was the effective ingredi-ent in the observed reductions.

49.   Frederiksen, L. W., Peterson, G. L., & Murphy, W. D. (1976). Controlled Smoking: Development and maintenance. Addictive Behaviors, 1, 193-196.

The goal of the study was to investigate controlled smoking with emphasis placed on smoking at or below a target rate set by the indi-vidual subject, rather then the techniques used to create the initial control. Sixteen subjects started treatment and gave a mean age of 22.75 years and mean smoking history of 25.06 cpd for 6.13 years.

Subjects were randomly assigned to one of two treatment groups. Half of the subjects were allocated to their first preference of treatment. The other half were allocated to their non-preferred treatment. All subjects self-monitored by recording the time they had started each cigarette during treatment, and estimated their smoking rate at follow-ups. A multiple-baseline research design across subjects was used. Half the subjects in each group began treatment after 1 week of baseline monitoring while the other half after 2 weeks of baseline monitoring. Programmed delay treatment (PD) involved the introduction of a temporal delay (specified by the experimenter) between removing the cigarette from the packet and actually lighting the cigarette. The time delay required the subject to review the reasons for and against smoking the cigarette. Contingency Contracting (CC) involved devising and signing a contract, which involved positive reinforcement (receiving a desired object or activity when smoking at or below the target rate).

Fifty percent of subjects in the PD group discontinued participation before the fourth week of the treatment. Chi-square analysis indicated attrition was not significantly related to either treatment preference or therapist. Analysis of smoking rates over treatment and follow-up indicated that PD did not produce the control found with CC. At end of treatment, PD smoked at their target rates 0% of the time while CC smoked at their target rates 62.5% of the time. Maintenance of controlled smoking was superior in CC subjects than PD subjects. However, smoking rate at follow-up was 50% or less than their initial smoking rate in 5 of the 7 CC subjects, but was still higher than the target rate. It was concluded that controlled smoking was a viable alternative to abstinence and CC procedure was superior to PD.

50.   Conway, J.B. (1977). Behavioral self-control of smoking through aversive conditioning and self-management. Journal of Consulting and Clinical Psychology, 45 (3), 348-357.

Ninety subjects completed pre-treatment smoking records and contract signing. Twenty more subjects were solicited via telephone for a no-apply control group. Ninety percent of subjects were undergraduates with a mean age of 21.1 years and mean smoking history of 19.37 cpd for 5.4 years. Subjects were organized into 10 groups and treatments were randomly assigned. All subjects kept daily smoking records for one week pre-treatment, three weeks of treatment and two follow-up weeks (following the 8th and 20th week post-treatment). A subject-nominated witness checked the smoking records. Six treatment sessions were held during three weeks. Half the subjects in each aversive conditioning group received self-management training in the form of a handbook and guidance by a therapist during the six treatment sessions. Half the subjects in the no aversive conditioning group received no treatment. The other half received the self-management training alone. Placebo shock group received a sub-threshold electric shock. They were told they couldn't feel it but it would reduce their urges to smoke. The therapist delivered shock group followed traditional aversive conditioning procedures where electric shocks were delivered to subjects by a therapist at a "barely tolerable" level. Subjects delivered shock group administered an electric shock to themselves following the therapists instructions. In the Imagined aversive group, a therapist verbally delivered aversive scenes which the subjects imagined. No apply control group were contacted by telephone and gave a smoking estimate pre-treatment and at both follow-ups but did not self-monitor or receive any treatment. Results found the rate of return to baseline smoking levels followed essentially the same trend for all treatments. No differences were found across the aversive conditioning groups. The authors discussed the clinically disappointing results where no treatment conditions resulted in maintained reductions across follow-ups. They suggested this result supported skepticism about the use of electrical aversion for smoking.

51.   Katz, R. C., Heiman, M., & Gordon, S. (1977). Effects of two self-management approaches on cigarette smoking. Addictive Behaviors, 2, 113-119.

A comparison between habit reversal and cognitive self-control for the treatment of smoking was presented. Thirty subjects attended a pre-treatment meeting which involved information about the program, collection of a refundable $25 deposit, signed consent form and smoking history questionnaire and distribution of a portable wrist counter to use when self-monitoring. Subjects self-monitored for one week baseline, and 14 weeks of treatment and follow-up, and reports were checked with "significant others". Subjects were randomly assigned to three treatment groups with mean baseline measures of 40 years of age, 5.2 motivation to quit rating, 156 cigarettes per week and 24.4 smoking years. Group 1 received habit reversal training involving aspects of understanding motivation, awareness training, competing response training, and public display procedure. Group 2 received cognitive self-control training, which involved self-instruction and self-reinforcement techniques. Group 3 was the patient education and will power control group. They received anti-smoking handouts and viewed anti-smoking films but were not presented with specific techniques for smoking control. Booster sessions staggered over three months post-treatment were made available but were not compulsory.

Results showed smoking decreased from baseline for all groups with no overall differences between them. Mean baseline smoking rates of between 50% and 60% were measured at follow-up. Twenty-seven percent were abstinent and only 20% of subjects returned to baseline levels of smoking. It was concluded that both habit reversal and self-instruction/self-reinforcement training produced rapid and sometimes permanent changes in smoking without using aversive techniques.

52.   Lamontagne, Y., Gagnon, M. A., Trudel, G., & Boisvert, J. M. (1978). Thought-stopping as a treatment for reducing cigarette smoking. The International Journal of the Addictions, 13 (2), 297-305.

Sixty-four male subjects with a mean age of 31.4 years and a mean smoking history of 27.3 cpd for 17.9 years were involved in the study. Two therapists delivered four treatments. Self-monitoring (C) recorded every cigarette smoked on a wrist counter. Subjects were told to reduce smoking using their own means. Badge-wearing group (B) wore a badge saying "I don't smoke" to decrease social influences and self-monitored their smoking as in (C) group. The group discussion (GD) contained six, 30-minute sessions in the first two weeks followed by four sessions in the last two weeks. The therapist led the debates in the general directions of tobacco problems and methods for reduction. Thought-stopping group (TS) met for an equivalent time to the GD group. Thought-stopping techniques were presented by tape-recorder. Subjects were encouraged to practice the techniques in real situations outside the sessions. The results showed that TS was the only group to give significantly different results from the others. It was reported that B subjects did not regularly wear the badge and this intervention was not more effective than C. Self-monitoring was considered a therapeutic tool and therefore did not serve as a "no treatment" control group. The GD group produced stable reduction during the treatment period but relapsed to near baseline by follow-up. The TS group was reluctant at first (they described the procedure as 'stupid') but produced and maintained large reductions from baseline, four of the six abstained during follow-up.

53.   Foxx, R. M., & Brown, R. A. (1979). Nicotine fading and self monitoring for cigarette abstinence or controlled smoking. Journal of Applied Behavior Analysis, 12, 111-125.

The aims of the study were to achieve a clinically significant percentage of abstainers and to reduce the tar/nicotine content of cigarettes in non-abstainers to a 'safer' level. Four treatment approaches were used: nicotine fading (by changing brands, not smoking rate)

(NF), self- monitoring (SM) (plotting daily intake of tar and nicotine), Nicotine fading and self-monitoring (NFSM), and a modified American Cancer Society Stop Smoking program (P) involving information to assist quitting followed by a 48 hour quit period. Forty-four subjects had a mean age of 31 years, and had smoked for an average of 14 years. All smoked at least one pack of cigarettes containing 0.7 mg of nicotine a day. The study included contract signing and reliability checks using significant others. At 18 month follow-up NFSM was the most successful intervention with 40% of subjects abstinent and a large reduction from baseline in daily intake of 61% nicotine and 70% tar in non-abstainers. Non-abstainers who achieved these reductions generally smoked less than baseline cpd. The NFSM group relapsed the least, followed by NF. SM group failed to produce significant abstinence or reductions. The P group showed a strong post-treatment effect, which deteriorated rapidly after the first month. The authors commented on why the NFSM was a more effective treatment, and about its superiority to aversive treatments.

54.   Colletti, G., & Supnick, J. A. (1980). Continued therapist contact as a maintenance strategy for smoking reduction. Journal of Consulting and Clinical Psychology, 48 (5), 665-667.

The effect of continued phone therapist contact was assessed using a non-aversive behavior based treatment package designed to reduce smoking. Twenty-nine subjects volunteered, and had a mean age of 41.03 years with a mean smoking history of 30.72 cpd for 22.81 years. The treatment package consisted of seven 1-hour sessions conducted in groups of five to ten people over a five-week period. Subjects self-monitored their smoking and suggestions for control techniques were presented. Subjects were randomly assigned to maintenance strategy, using continued therapist contact for four weeks or no maintenance strategy. After the four weeks all subjects were required to send in weekly smoking rates for three months, some subjects were reminded with a phone call. Twelve-month follow-up rates were obtained and verified by a CO reading. After treatment, subjects achieved a 76% reduction of the baseline rate. Results showed the experimental group had superior maintenance at six months. No significant difference between the groups was observed at 12 months (due to improvement by the control group rather than relapse by the experimental group). Most subjects maintained long-term smoking reduction.

55.   Raw, M., & Russell, M. A. (1980). Rapid smoking, cue exposure and support in the modification of smoking. Behavior Research and Therapy, 18 (5), 363-372.

Specific and nonspecific treatment effects were investigated by comparing rapid smoking, simple support and cue exposure. Forty-nine subjects from a hospital smokers clinic started treatment, had a mean age of 39.5 years and smoked an average of 34.9 cpd started treatment. Self-monitoring of smoking behavior lasted for six weeks, with treatment for three months. Cessation was encouraged from the first day of treatment. A follow-up session occurred six months post-treatment. Follow-up by mail occurred at three and 12 months post-treatment. Support treatment consisted of self-monitoring, encouragement, advice and support from the therapist and other group members. Cue exposure treatment consisted of support and practice in cue exposure to a range of different cues. Rapid smoking treatment consisted of support and inhaling a cigarette on command every 6 seconds, until they could tolerate no more. This was repeated twice after a five-minute break. A reduction of 58%, 74% and 55% was achieved post-treatment for support, cue exposure and rapid smoking respectively. Post-treatment differences between treatments at 3-, 6-, and 12-months follow-up were all not significant. Twenty-two percent was abstinent post-treatment, falling to 14% at 1 year with no significant differences between groups. A self-monitoring, self-control and treatment effect was observed and discussed. The results showed that neither rapid smoking nor cue exposure was more effective than simple support. Reasons for the lower success rate in this study compared to others included differences in subject population like age, baseline cigarette consumption, and degree of dependence.

56.   Foxx, R. M., Brown, R. M., & Katz, I. (1981). Nicotine fading and self monitoring for cigarette abstinence or controlled smoking: A two and one-half year follow-up. Behavior Therapist, 4 (2), 21-23.

A 30 month follow-up was presented on Foxx and Brown's 1979 study on nicotine fading and self-monitoring in the treatment of smoking to produce abstinence or controlled smoking. Four treatment conditions were compared: nicotine fading (NF) where subjects progressively changed brands to less nicotine and tar; self-monitoring (SM) where subjects plotted daily intake of nicotine and tar; combined nicotine fading and self-monitoring (NFSM); and a slightly modified version of the American Cancer Society Stop Smoking Program (ACS). At the 18-month follow-up results showed that NFSM was the most successful in maintaining an abstinence rate of 40%. Half the non-abstainers had reduced their smoking rate while the other half had increased. The NFSM group maintained daily nicotine and tar intake reductions of 61% and 70% respectively from baseline.

The 30-month follow-up was conducted by telephone and information was collected about average daily smoking rate, brand smoked and number of days abstinent.   Reliability of subjects' self-reports was checked by one of the significant others, and in all cases reports were verified.   The four abstainers in the NFSM group had maintained abstinence, with the addition of one non-abstainer who quit between the 18- and 30-month follow-up.   In the NF group, one abstainer remained abstinent while one had relapsed.   At 30-month follow-up, all non-abstainers in the NFSM and ACS groups had maintained reductions in tar and nicotine levels lower than baseline brands.   The NFSM group achieved the greatest percentage reductions.   Sixty percent of non-abstainers at 30-month follow-up were smoking fewer cigarettes than baseline.   The 30-month follow-up result showed that the NFSM group had continued to achieve both study goals; a clinically significant abstinence level and controlled 'safer' smoking for non-abstainers.

57.   Murray, R. G., & Hobbs, S. A. (1981). Effects of self-reinforcement and self-punishment in smoking reduction: Implications for broad-spectrum behavioral approaches. Addictive Behaviors, 6(1), 36-67.

The individual and combined effects of self-reinforcement and self-punishment in a smoking reduction program were investigated.   Forty-four subjects had a mean age of 27.4 years and smoked a mean of 26.6 cpd for 10.2 smoking years.   Subjects self-monitored smoking for one-week baseline, three weeks of treatment and one-week follow-up.   All subjects were given daily smoking reduction goals during treatment. The self-reinforcement (SR) group established a monetary reward for achieving the daily goals, which was spent on a tangible reward at the end of each week.   The self-punishment (SP) group agreed to forfeit money to a charity when reduction goals were not met.   The self-punishment plus self-reinforcement (SP+SR) group combined these procedures. The self-monitoring (SM) control group had no reinforce-ment or punishment.   Forty subjects completed the program.   All groups achieved reductions in the number of cigarettes smoked per day.   Results from post-treatment, 3-month and 3-year follow-up indicate that SP and SP+SR groups were significantly more effective than SR or SM groups.   The authors concluded that self-punishment should be included in broad-spectrum behavioral approaches to smoking reduction.

58.   Hills, A. A. (1982). Target setting and self-control for smoking. Psychological Reports, 50(1), 68-70.

Health Locus of Control and self or therapist setting of targets was assessed in the modification of cigarette smoking. Sixty subjects were selected from responses to a newspaper advertisement for volunteers. They had a mean age of 39.2 years and mean smoking history of 25.7 cpd for 21.6 smoking years. Subjects were telephoned at the end of each week for self-monitoring reports. They were placed on a new reduction target for the following week, selected either by himself or herself or by a therapist. A waiting list control group consisted of subjects who did not start the treatment program until first treatment group had finished treatment. Results showed that therapist-paced subjects achieved a greater reduction maintained at 3-month follow-up than self-paced subjects. Analysis of variance showed no significant differences between the 2 treatments, between the acceptance ratings for the treatments or between the accuracy of instruction completion by subjects in the treatments. As in other studies, a stuck point was found at about 10-12 cpd. Locus of control data did not show any significant differences. Replication recommendations were discussed.

59.   Newman, A., & Bloom, R. (1982). Smoking reduction: A comparison of the effectiveness of rapid smoking and increasing delay training. Addictive Behaviors, 7(1), 93-96.

The experiment was designed to compare the effectiveness of rapid smoking and increasing delay training in the self-control of smoking behavior. Twenty undergraduate volunteer subjects smoked a minimum of 30 cpd for more than one year and completed self-monitoring for seven days pre- and post-treatment, and a 2-hour experimental session for five days. Treatment consisted of a pre-test and post-test. Electrodes were placed on the index and fourth finger. Subjects were asked to light a cigarette and put it in an ashtray and wait as long as possible before taking another puff. Three self-control trials were completed and the subjects' delay tolerance recorded. Treatment consisted of either increasing delay (where the delay between puffs increased 10 seconds on every trial) or rapid smoking (where subjects took a puff every 10 seconds during the session). Increasing delay training resulted in superior self-control than rapid smoking on a resistance to temptation task. Although smoking reductions across treatments were equivalent, the authors suggested that increasing delay training should make it easier for subjects to withstand the urges to smoke.

60.   Glasgow, R. E., Kleges, R. C., Godding, P. R., & Gegelman, R. (1983). Controlled smoking, with or without carbon monoxide

feedback, as an alternative for chronic smokers. Behavior Therapy, 14 (3), 386-397.

Controlled smoking consisted of a complex treatment package designed to reduce cigarette smoking without elimination by modifying the smoking response dimensions of substance, rate and topography. Sixty chronic cigarette smokers averaged 41 years, smoked an average of 35 cpd for 22 years and were unable or unwilling to quit but wished to reduce their smoking. Subjects were randomly assigned to one of three treatment conditions. Controlled smoking (CS) was designed to achieve 50% reductions in nicotine content, daily consumption, and percentage of each cigarette smoked. Controlled smoking plus carbon monoxide (CO) feedback (CS+CO) received the same treatment as CS but also received CO assessment and feedback at the beginning of each treatment session. The waiting list controls (C) were informed of a delay of five weeks before treatment. Following the delay the C group received the CS treatment plus feedback on the amount of nicotine consumed daily to investigate whether CO feedback or any kind of feedback was effective.

One way analysis of covariance at post-test revealed highly significant treatment effects on all measures. CS consistently produced meaningful reductions in smoking behavior, maintained adequately for at least six months. Few differences were found on behavioral measures between CS and CS+CO. The additional time and expense of providing CO feedback may not be warranted (also supported by results from the nicotine consumption feedback). Although no evidence of compensatory smoking on the self-monitoring measures were reported, CO reductions were not as great as expected. This may indicate some compensation. Subjects were successful in reducing nicotine content but less successful in achieving the 50% reductions in daily cigarette consumption and percentage of each cigarette smoked. Limitations of this study and future research were discussed.

61.   Glasgow, R. E., Klesges, R. C., Godding, P. R., Vasey, M. W., & O'Neill, K. (1984). Evaluation of a worksite-controlled smoking program. Journal of Consulting and Clinical Psychology, 52 (1), 137-138.

The authors conducted a controlled smoking program in an occupational setting (a telephone company) for smokers who wished to quit or to reduce their smoking. Thirty-six subjects averaged 37 years and had a mean estimated smoking history of 30 cpd for 18 years. Subjects were randomly assigned to three conditions, abrupt reduction (A), gradual reduction (G) or gradual reduction plus feedback (GF). All treatments altered nicotine content, percentage of cigarette smoked and the number of cigarettes smoked. Subjects in all conditions were able to alter each of the target behaviors and maintained changes at six month follow-up without evidence of "compensatory smoking" in measured CO levels. The G group was more effective in producing long-term cessation than the abrupt reduction condition. The addition of feedback was not significantly better than abrupt reduction or gradual reduction alone.

62.   Glasgow, R. E., Klesges, R. C., Klesges, L. M., Vasey, M. W., & Gunnarson, D. F. (1985). Long-term effects of a controlled smoking program: A 2-½ year follow-up. Behavior Therapy, 16, 303-307.

A 2-½ year follow-up is reported on a study involving 48 chronic smokers who wished to reduce (but not quit) smoking. Participants completed one of three treatments. Basic controlled smoking (CS) involved sequential 50% reductions in nicotine content, frequency of smoking and percent of each cigarette smoked. The second group was controlled smoking plus weekly carbon monoxide feedback (CS+CO). The third group was "delayed controlled smoking" treatment with feedback on daily nicotine levels (C). At six month follow-up both CS and CS+CO groups achieved significantly greater reductions in each of the target behaviors than the C group. The two groups were not significantly different from each other. Subjects were contacted 2 ½ years post-treatment. Information was obtained for all 48 subjects, although only 28 attended an interview. Although non-abstinent subjects generally smoked more at the 2-½ year follow-up, levels were still significantly less than baseline on all dependent variables. The authors concluded that relatively permanent reductions in smoking behavior could be achieved by some heavy smokers. In particular, reductions in nicotine content and CO levels achieved superior maintenance than reductions in percentage of each cigarette smoked.

63.   Hatsukami, D. K., Dahlgren, L., Zimmerman, R., & Hughes, J. R. (1988). Symptoms of tobacco withdrawal from total cigarette cessation versus partial cigarette reduction. Psychopharmacology, 94, 242-247.

The severity of acute tobacco withdrawal symptoms between total cigarette abstinence and 2 types of partial cigarette reductions were analyzed. Thirty-two subjects averaged 24.2 years of age, 26 cpd of 0.88-mg nicotine for 7.3 years, with 3.5 quitting attempts and were paid $50 to meet with experimental conditions. Subjects were randomly assigned into three groups, total cessation (C), 50%

reduction in smoking rate (Rc), or reduction in nicotine yield of cigarettes (Rn). All subjects attended laboratory sessions for eight days. Subjects smoked at their normal rate for the first three sessions and then according to their group specifications for the next five sessions. They were asked to abstain from alcohol and maintain caffeine intake throughout the study. Abstinence and reductions were verified through carbon monoxide and saliva cotinine samples. Heart rate, body weight, Profile of Mood States (POMS), Stanford Sleep Scale, and a withdrawal symptoms checklist by self and a significant other were collected at each session.

The effects of the two partial reduction procedures were remarkably similar with no significant differences on any scale. C group showed significantly greater decreased heart rate, and increased weight, number of awakenings during sleep, total score on the self-rated and observer-rated withdrawal symptom checklist, and anger/hostility on the POMS. The results showed that withdrawal symptoms appeared within 24 hours for all measures of the C group, and showed more withdrawal than Rc or Rn on all significant measures. The authors concluded that for smokers not trying to quit, partial reductions of tobacco did not result in more severe withdrawal symptoms than subjects who stopped entirely.

64.   Buchkremer, G., Bents, H., Horstmann, M., Opitz, K., & Tolle, R. (1989). Combination of behavioral smoking cessation with transdermal nicotine substitution. Addictive Behaviors, 14, 229-238.

The study was designed to investigate whether transdermal nicotine substitution could significantly enhance the effectiveness of self-controlled smoking reduction. One hundred and thirty-one smokers were randomly assigned to three treatment conditions. The control group (C) received behavioral training in self-control of cigarette reduction. In addition to behavioral training, the nicotine plaster group (N) received self-adhesive patches containing a changing dosage of nicotine. These patches were worn continuously for the duration of the experiment on the back, upper arm, or thigh. The patches were changed each morning. The third group received the behavioral training and wore placebo patches (P), which were indistinguishable from the nicotine patches. Behavioral training included gradual reduction of cigarette consumption, increase in cognitive dissonance, control of smoking situations, contract management and relapse pre-vention. N subjects were found to reduce smoking significantly more rapidly then P or C subjects. The proportion of abstinent subjects was significantly higher in the N group than the P and C groups. It was concluded that transdermal nicotine substitution was an ideal supplement to behavior modification methods for smoking cessation.

65.   Glasgow, R. E., Morray, K., & Lichtenstein, E. (1989). Controlled smoking versus abstinence as a treatment goal: The hopes and fears may be unfounded. Behavior Therapy, 20 (1), 77-91.

The first goal of the study was to assess whether the abstinence-based program produced higher cessation rates. The second goal was to determine whether the cessation reduction program produced greater reductions in smoking behavior and carbon monoxide (CO) levels among subjects not achieving abstinence. Underlying theories and previous research of controlled smoking were reviewed in detail. Sixty-six smokers averaged 39.6 years and had a mean smoking history of 26 cpd for 21 years. No mention of a controlled smoking option was made during recruitment. Subjects were randomly assigned to one of two treatment conditions. The abstinence-based condition (AB) had three sessions preparation (subjects target individual cigarettes to eliminate to gain experience coping with non-smoking in particular situations), quitting on the fourth session. The next three sessions emphasized relapse prevention. Cessation controlled smoking condition (CCS) encouraged subjects to quit. If abstinence was not achievable, smoking reduction was acceptable. The first three sessions led to successive changes in the smoking rate. Session 4 gave the option of quitting or further changes in smoking topography (by reducing the percentage of each cigarette smoked). The last 2 sessions were concerned with maintenance, goal setting and assessment. The only between-group difference on pre-treatment characteristics was nicotine content of cigarette brand smoked, which was significantly higher for CCS subjects.

Twenty-one percent of subjects failed to complete post-test evaluations. It was found they smoked significantly more cigarettes, scored higher on the Fagerstrom Tolerance Scale and had higher CO levels at baseline. Post-treatment subjects reported abstinence rates of 52% and 70% for AS and CCS respectively. Non-abstinent subjects in both groups achieved significant reductions. There were no significant differences between abstainers and non-abstainers at 6-month follow-up for either group. It was concluded that long-term cessation rates for CCS were comparable to AB. CCS failed to produce greater reductions among non-abstainers than AB. The optimistic claims for the effects of controlled smoking were not supported.

66.   Price, J. H., Krol, R. A., Desmond, S. M., Losh, D. P., Roberts, S. M.,
      & Snyder, F. F. (1991). Comparison of three antismoking
      interventions among pregnant women in an urban setting: A
      randomized trial. Psychological Reports, 68 (2), 595-604.

One hundred and nine female pregnant (less than 28 weeks at the start
of the study) subjects completed the study. They had a mean age of
22.6 years; most were single (58%), white (70%) and unemployed
(81%) with 87% not graduating from high school. Only subjects who
blew 8 ppm of CO or higher were considered smokers and included in
the study. Subjects completed a questionnaire and were randomly
assigned (by the toss of a die) to one of three groups (resulting in
uneven groups). Educational videotape group (V) watched a 6½-
minute videotape about health risks to the unborn baby and about
benefits if maternal cigarette smoking was stopped. A pamphlet on
"how to stop smoking" was also distributed. One month later a second
four-minute video was viewed with information from the first video as
well as methods of cessation. American Lung Association Group
(ALA) received a booklet titled "Freedom from smoking for you and
your baby" and were given a brief overview and explanation. The
booklet emphasized behavior modification skills, relaxation techniques, and supports from significant others. A second session after
one month reviewed progress and answered questions. Physicians
Advice group (C) received usual advice from physicians about the
implications of smoking while pregnant. This advice was not
uniformly structured, but varied from physician to physician. Two to
three weeks prior to delivery the questionnaire was completed again
with a carbon monoxide reading.

Forty-three percent of subjects reduced the number of cigarettes
smoked, 6% quit and 49% continued at the same rate. The three intervention programs were equally effective in assisting reduction, with no
significant difference between the amount of reduction. The mean
reduction was small, ranging form 2.3 to 4.3 cpd. The large dropout
rate and the demographics of this sample, compared to other studies
were discussed.

67.   Salkovskis, P. M., & Reynolds, M. (1993). Thought suppression and
      smoking cessation. Behavior Research and Therapy, 32(2), 193-201.

The study was designed to evaluate three questions. Do people who
attempt to reduce their smoking try to suppress thoughts of smoking?
Does experimentally-increased thought suppression of naturally-
occurring "smoking thoughts" produce enhancement and /or rebound

effects on those thoughts? Does a simple distraction task assist people in thought suppression without enhancing rebound effects? Sixty-two smokers participated, who were committed to reduction or cessation of smoking. Participants were allocated into three groups, Suppression (S, n=22, mean age=35.3), Mention (M, n=20, mean age=38.3), and Distraction (D, n=20, mean age=38.1). All subjects completed a questionnaire about smoking-related intrusive thoughts, STAI (state form), and also rated their tension and relaxation. The number of thoughts during the target period was counted on a hand-held counter. The questionnaire of intrusive thoughts and cognitions, STAI (state and trait forms), and Beck Anxiety and Depression Inventories were completed post-test. Smoking-related thoughts occurred frequently and intensely in people trying to reduce or quit smoking. These people also tried to suppress their smoking-related thoughts. A simple distraction task plus relaxation were found to be highly successful in reducing the frequency of intrusive thoughts. The study suggested that the "think of something else" advice that people who attempt to reduce or stop smoking are often given is inappropriate, unless it is used with a specific and structured distracter. In addition, specific instructions on how to divert attention from smoking-related thoughts are also effective in reducing intrusive thoughts.

68.   Spanos, N. P., Mondoux, T. J., & Burgess, C. A. (1995). Comparison of multi-component hypnotic and non-hypnotic treatments for smoking.   Special Issue: To the memory of Nicholas Spanos. Contemporary Hypnosis, 12(1), 12-19.

The objectives of the study were to compare the effectiveness of hypnotic and non-hypnotic treatment when multiple strategies for smoking cessation were presented. Active hypnotic and non-hypnotic smoking cessation treatments were compared with a placebo treatment. Fifty-four volunteer subjects aged between 19 and 62 years were recruited through newspaper advertisements. They were randomly assigned to one of four conditions: hypnotic treatment (H), non-hypnotic treatment (NH), placebo (P), or no-treatment control (C). Subjects in the C group were told they were on a waiting list and would be administered treatment following three months of self-monitoring.   Subjects in the three treatment groups self-monitored smoking for two weeks baseline, then attended two, 1-hour treatment sessions and were tested for hypnotizability. The H group received a 10-minute hypnotic induction procedure. This was followed by various hypnotic procedures to reduce their cravings and urges for cigarettes allowing abstinence.   The NH group received the same treatment excluding the hypnotic induction; the procedures were labelled "cognitive restructuring" instead of hypnosis. The P group was informed that subliminal messages could reduce their urge to smoke and were told to listen to an audiotape of music containing subliminal messages (the music did not contain subliminal messages).

All three groups were given a 15-minute audiocassette with a shortened version of their treatment for daily playback. Therapists contacted subjects during a 3-month follow-up period. Nine subjects withdrew from the study. Analysis of variance (excluding dropouts) showed that H and NH conditions did not vary in the number of cigarettes they smoked across the five intervals. There was a significant decrease, which had returned to baseline levels at follow-up. One subject reduced smoking by 50% and two subjects by 25% (all from the H group) by the last follow-up. The failure to find significant correlations between treatment outcome and hypnotizability was discussed.

3

MULTIPLE TREATMENTS

69.   Ober, D. C. (1968). Modification of smoking behavior. Journal of
       Consulting and Clinical Psychology, 32, 543-549.

Sixty subjects were selected from a volunteer group of 79 students. The
smoking criteria were inhalation of more than 20 cpd for more than a
year, and a desire to stop smoking. Groups of 15 students were randomly assigned to one of three treatment groups, or a no-treatment
control group. Each of the treatment subjects was randomly assigned
to one of two therapists. All treatment subjects received a treatment
manual, a habit breaker, and then completed ten treatment sessions.
The self-control group's habit breaker was a card saying, "I have the
self-control not to smoke this cigarette" which was read each time a
cigarette was desired. The self-control program included basic principles of learning applied to smoking behavior, consequences of smoking, and an analysis of behavior and application of the self-control
principles.

The aversion group's habit breaker was a smaller aversive stimulator
that delivered a self-administered shock. The level of the shock was
changed at each meeting to a level described by the subject as 'pain-
ful'. The shock was self-administered with each craving. Shocks continued until the desire for a cigarette could not be postponed. Again
principles of a learning approach and consequences of smoking
behavior were included. The transactional analysis program's habit
breaker was a card saying "I don't have to play the smoking game".
The card was read each time a cigarette was desired. Several smoking
games were devised and played, with an emphasis on reasons for

smoking. Topics covered included the principles of a transactional analysis, the reason for playing the games, the structure, and some examples of the games. Analysis of variance found no effect differentiating therapists or type of treatment. Type of treatment (independent of which kind) was found to be highly effective, with a mean reduction from 25 cpd to 7 cpd at 1-month follow-up. The authors concluded that self-control of smoking behavior could be established.

70.   Levinson, B. L., Shapiro, D., Schwartz, G. E., & Tursky, B. (1971). Smoking elimination by gradual reduction. Behavior Therapy, 2, 477-487.

The focus of the study was to test the efficacy of a signalling device to reduce the reported incidence of situational cues in smoking behavior. The difference between using three and one group meetings, and between using a timer versus a counter as the signalling device in eliminating smoking behavior was assessed. Fifty-two subjects who smoked between 30 and 45 cpd were divided into four groups matched for age, gender and smoking rate. Subjects in groups 1 and 2 were given a timer. They were instructed to only smoke one cigarette whenever the timer sounded (whether they wanted to or not), but not to smoke at any other time. The timers were set with a scheduled quota of 32 cigarettes per 16-hour day for the first week. The quota was then systematically reduced to 14 cpd in week 6 and abstinence in week 12. Subjects in groups 3 and 4 used a golf counter to record each cigarette smoked. They were told not to smoke above the quota described for groups 1 and 2.

All subjects completed questionnaires about smoking habits at the initial meeting and at 8-week, 12-week, and 3-month follow-up. Subjects in groups 2 and 4 attended a meeting after week 8 and 12 to complete questionnaires. The subjects discussed problems, while subjects in groups 1 and 3 received questionnaires by post. More than half the subjects withdrew from (or did not complete) the program. More subjects in the timer condition did not complete than in the counter condition. Subjects in the timer condition were more successful in abstinence at 3-month follow-up than the counter condition. Subjects in group meeting condition who completed the program reported greater confidence of success in quitting than subjects in groups 1 and 3. Most subjects were not able to reduce below 12 cpd. A pattern of "stuck points" was found at 24.6 cpd, 13.1 cpd and 12.0 cpd. At these points subjects reported difficulty and some stopped the program. It was concluded that the timer condition, although more difficult, may have reduced the situational cues to smoke, and therefore produced more successful reductions. A "stuck point" may exist around 12 cpd where further reductions are difficult. This suggest additional therapeutic measures are required to make further reductions to achieve abstinence.

71.   Marston, A. R., & McFall, R. M. (1971). Comparison of behavior modification approaches to smoking reduction. Journal of Consulting and Clinical Psychology, 36(2), 153-162.

Two experimental treatments and two control conditions were compared for the modification of cigarette smoking. Minimal treatment control conditions were used instead of no-treatment control. The authors claimed the critical test of an experimental treatment efficacy was to reduce smoking significantly more than minimal treatment procedures. Therefore a minimal treatment control is an appropriate baseline for treatment comparison. Sixty-five undergraduate subjects had a mean age of 20.9 years and mean smoking history of 25.9 cpd for 4½ years . The stimulus satiation condition had three phases, satiation (smoking three times the normal rate), reduction, and maintained abstinence. Subjects were required to follow five rules that altered the usual routines and habits of smoking during all phases. In the hierarchical reduction condition, smoking was reduced gradually in 4 consecutive time periods of each day. Abstinence during the easiest time period of the waking day was achieved first, and then other time periods, until total abstinence had occurred. Counter-conditioning techniques such as relaxation were presented to aid reduction. The pill-control condition used a non-drug aversive spice tablet (Pronicotyl). The pill coated the mouth with a herb compound producing an aversive taste when smoking. Subjects sucked a pill before, during and after each cigarette. "Cold turkey control" group was told to quit on their own. They were given printed material that suggested helpful hints on how to stop.

Each of the conditions showed its own characteristic reduction curve, achieving a mean reduction of 25% of baseline post-treatment. There was a marked relapse by all groups at follow-up. There was a failure to obtain significant post-treatment between-group differences. The level of smoking reductions reported post-treatment were paired with high rates of relapse. This was described as a replication of most past research. A significant therapist effect was found. This indicated the importance in avoiding single-therapist designs. An analysis of the curves that described the subjects' response rate during treatment demonstrated that the different therapeutic strategies in each condition were significantly different in shape.

72.   Gordon, S. B., & Hall, L. A. (1973). Therapy determined by
       assessment in the modification of smoking: A case study. Journal of
       Behavior Therapy and Experimental Psychiatry, 4, 379-382.

A case study designed to show the effectiveness of a client matching
therapeutic technique on controlling smoking behavior was presented.
A woman aged 52 suffering from smoking-related illnesses reported a
smoking history of 30 cpd for 36 years. The subject self-monitored
smokes throughout the study. Smoking was restricted to a limited
range of stimulus conditions excluding pleasurable activities for the
first 2 sessions. The subject had reported that heavy smoking reduced
the pleasurable taste. Rapid smoking was provided from session 3 to
11. Results showed during initiation of self-control procedures, a
large reduction occurred. This was maintained over 10 days. Rapid
smoking produced gradual reductions toward total abstinence. Follow-
up at three-months indicated smoking reductions were maintained to
one or two cigarettes per week. At 6-month follow-up the subject had
relapsed to 13 cpd, which was attributed to depression following
medical treatment. She reported deterioration in the taste of cigarettes.
The authors emphasize the importance of accurate assessment to
match the treatment to the client. Control of variables in specific
interventions, and continued contact following treatment termination
was also emphasized.

73.   St. Pierre, R., & Lawrence, P. S. (1975). Reducing smoking using
       positive self-management. Journal of School Health, 45 (1), 7-9.

The study was designed to reduce the smoking behavior of students by
combining a variety of behavioral techniques developed to alter
smoking level. Previous cognitive approaches from teaching students
which emphasized the adverse effects of smoking and hoped for a subsequent change in behavior had proved unsuccessful. Forty-five subjects were assigned to one of two treatment groups. The remainder
were placed in a no-treatment control group. The aversive treatment
group was given techniques emphasizing the negative consequences of
smoking. The positive treatment group was given techniques emphasizing positive elements associated with smoking reduction. After
treatment, subjects were assigned to either a positive maintenance
group, aversive maintenance group or no maintenance control group.
Positive treatment and maintenance made use of peer reinforcement
using a buddy system. Participants read a list of positive outcomes,
kept a diary of smoking behavior, used self-rewards and signed contracts. Aversive treatment and maintenance consisted of films stress-

ing harmful effects of smoking, role-playing fear, noticing unpleasant effects of smoking in others and satiation techniques.

At 3-month follow-up all subjects who received positive treatment, irrespective of maintenance, reduced smoking level by 50%. Subjects who received positive maintenance, irrespective of treatment also achieved a 50% rate reduction. Students who received both positive treatment and maintenance achieved reductions of 57%. The largest reduction of 60% occurred in the group that received aversive treatment, followed by positive maintenance. The group which was most like programs in previous health education campaigns (aversive treatment followed by no maintenance) had the poorest reduction of only 19%. Use of techniques by students in their natural environment was discussed.

74.   Delahunt, J., & Curran, J. P. (1976). Effectiveness of negative practice and self-control techniques in the reduction of smoking behavior. Journal of Consulting and Clinical Psychology, 44 (6), 1002-1007.

Fifty female subjects had an average age of 27.9 years and mean smoking history of 25.27 cpd for 9.84 years. At the preliminary meeting, subjects completed questionnaires including demographic details, smoking history, Eysenck Personality Inventory and Internal-External Locus of Control Scale. Subjects were informed how to monitor and record their smoking behavior. Each of the four treatment groups met for six 1-hour sessions over three weeks. The non-specific condition group was told to quit "cold turkey". They had group discussions and support with therapist contact but received no specific treatment designed to reduce smoking. The negative practice group included non-specific conditions, and they engaged in negative practice of smoking behavior between the third and fourth sessions. The self-control group were given various strategies of self-control, with reward/punishment and assistance from the therapist and group discussions. The combination practice group was given instructions on both negative practice and self-control strategies. A significant difference in abstinence data between the control and combined treatment groups was found. This illustrated the superiority of the combined treatment group. The results also showed that negative practice and self-control groups produced similar results in both reductions and abstinence. Combined treatment was superior in both measures.

75.   Lando, H. A. (1977). Successful treatment of smokers with a broadspectrum behavioral approach. Journal of Consulting and Clinical psychology, 45, 361-366.

The study compared a broad-spectrum treatment with a short-term control, against a goal to eliminate cigarette smoking. Thirty-four subjects had a mean age of 31.2 years, a mean smoking history of 28.7 cpd for 12.4 years. Subjects were randomly assigned to conditions. All subjects attended six, 45-minute sessions over one week. Twenty-five minutes were spent on aversive conditioning (continuous smoking). Subjects were encouraged to smoke as much as possible on their own between sessions. Control subjects were told to abstain after the initial week of aversive conditioning, and to maintain abstinence on their own. Experimental subjects attended seven maintenance sessions with group discussion and contract signing in the two months after the initial week of aversive conditioning. The contracts had several elements including forfeiting money for every cigarette smoked, specific rewards for abstinence, and punishments for smoking. Booster treatment sessions of rapid smoking followed any relapse of smoking.

Experimental subjects reported 100% reduction after the initial week of aversive conditioning, compared to 90% reduction for the control group. At 6-month follow-up, experimental subjects had maintained an 81% reduction from baseline. The control group had relapsed to 44% reduction from baseline. A two way ANOVA found significant main effects for condition, and time, and a significant interaction for condition X time. At 6-month follow-up 76% of experimental subjects remained abstinent. Only 35% remained abstinent in the control group. The authors suggested that abstinence was a more meaningful criterion of treatment effects than percentage reductions. Most smokers were apparently unable to permanently maintain significantly reduced smoking levels. The authors also suggest that the goal of most subjects in treatment is abstinence. Group cohesiveness, adequate controls and the need to apply research in clinical settings were discussed.

76.   Barbarin, O. A. (1978). Comparison of symbolic and overt aversion in the self-control of smoking. Journal of Consulting and Clinical Psychology, 46 (6), 1569-1571.

The study compared rapid smoking, covert sensitization and its combination for reduced or eliminated smoking. Sixty subjects with a mean age of 40 had all smoked at least 1 pack a day. Subjects were assigned to one of three experimental groups or to a control group. Baseline smoking was measured and treatment was given in the form of training in ten, 1-hour sessions over one month. The rapid smoking group was required to smoke every six seconds until they could no longer tolerate it. The covert sensitization group imagined aversive consequences from smoking and also positive refusal to smoke. The combination group learned both rapid smoking and covert sensitization procedures. The control group was sent descriptions of self-control procedures used in the program and was contacted by telephone weekly for one month and also at follow-up points to monitor their progress. Significant differences were found in smoking rates between each experimental group and the control group. The rapid smoking group achieved greater reductions than covert sensitization. There was no significant difference between the combined treatment and either treatment alone, even at 1-year follow-up. The authors concluded that while rapid smoking appeared superior in both reductions and abstinence, covert sensitization showed promise as a self-modification procedure for controlled smoking.

77. Elliot, C. H., & Denney, D. R. (1978). A multiple-component treatment approach to smoking reduction. Journal of Consulting and Clinical Psychology, 46 (6), 1330-1339.

Sixty-three subjects had an average age of 29.4 years and average smoking history of 27.0 cpd for 12.4 years. A pre-test session involved completion of smoking history, the name of a close friend (for accuracy check) and semantic differential scale questionnaires. A week of normal smoking and butt collection was encouraged, to determine baseline values. The subjects were divided into four groups. The untreated group collected butts and were involved in pre-test, post-test and follow-up sessions. They were told to quit via their own efforts. The non-specific group received lectures, educational material and mild encouragement, followed by data collection and a 45-minute non-directive group discussion. The rapid smoking group received the non-specific procedure plus two rapid smoking trials each session. The package treatment group received the non-specific procedure plus rapid smoking, applied relaxation, covert sensitization, systematic desensitization, self-reward/punishment, cognitive restructuring, behavioral rehearsal and emotional role playing. At the post-test session, subjects handed in butts from the previous week and completed the semantic differential scale again. Subjects were randomly divided into three booster conditions. They were given three additional booster sessions before the 3-month follow-up. The differences in percentage of baseline between conditions were explained by the number of abstainers. The package group showed more abstainers than the other three conditions. The booster sessions found no reliable effects. The authors concluded that controlled smoking procedures incorporated in the package treatment would aid smokers who did not wish to quit improving their overall success.

78.   Glasgow, R. E. (1978). Effects of a self-control manual, rapid smoking, and amount of therapist contact on smoking reduction. Journal of Consulting and Clinical Psychology, 46(6), 1439-1447.

The study evaluated a self-help treatment manual with instructions on stimulus control, rapid smoking and coping relaxation techniques. Sixty-two subjects had an average of 32.6 years and a mean smoking history of 24.7 cpd for 15.1 years.   The subjects were randomly assigned to one of four treatment groups. Minimal contact self-control group (MC) was given a 37-page treatment manual with progress recorded on a schedule. Subjects watched a demonstration of relaxa-tion procedures by a therapist. Subjects had more contact with the therapist to receive the first rapid smoking session.   Weekly phone calls to report progress was the only other contact with the therapist. High contact self-control group (HC) received the same manual as MC but also had seven meetings with the therapist over three weeks. This contact assisted implementation of assignments in each section.   High contact rapid smoking group (RS) was the same as the MC group. All sessions however were administered by a therapist with the first 9 days a preparation period (instead of stimulus control and relaxation). High contact normal paced smoking group (NS) received an aversive smoking procedure with the same rationale, number and spacing of sessions and procedures to RS group.   At 6-month follow-up, 16% (compared to 40% 1 week post-treatment) were abstinent and subjects averaged 70.4% (compared to 16.7% 1 week post-treatment) of base-line cpd.   The results showed only moderate effectiveness; groups showed no significant difference and thus high therapist contact may not be warranted.

79.   Johnson, E. K., & Chamberlain, J. M. (1978). The treatment of smoking as a self-defeating behavior. Journal of Psychology, 98 (1), 37-43.

A Workshop for Eliminating Self-Defeating Behaviors (ESDB) was utilized as a self-control treatment to alter cigarette smoking.   The workshop identified how self-defeating behavior (SDB) started. Subjects assumed responsibility for SDB, identified the cost and choices in continuing SDB, techniques used in maintaining and fears in living without SDB. Finally subjects faced their fears.   The Rotter Internal-External Locus of Control scale and a smoking questionnaire was completed by 18 subjects who smoked a mean of 23.6 cpd and gave a mean score of 7.3 on the I-E scale.   A significant reduction in daily smoking was reported for the experimental group (23 to 9 cpd). They also reported a significant change from external to internal locus of control post-treatment. At follow-up (4 weeks post-treatment) the change in locus of control had returned to external with similar scores to pre-treatment. No significant relapse in smoking was reported. The ESDB workshop was effective in helping smokers achieve significant reductions in smoking behavior maintained at a 4-week follow-up.

80.   Kaplan, G. D., & Cowles, A. (1978). Health locus of control and health value in the prediction of smoking reduction. Health Education Monographs, 6 (2), 129-137.

Health Locus of Control (HLC) and a measure of health values (THV) were analyzed in a smoking reduction study to assess the predictiveness of social learning theory in smoking reduction. Thirty-one subjects with a mean age of 37.0 years and mean smoking history of 23 cpd for 17.7 years completed a study in 3 phases. Phase 1 had completion of research questionnaires including HLC and THV scales and seven weekly small group multiple component treatment sessions. This included rapid smoking, self-monitoring, self-control training and cognitive behavior modification training. Gradual reduction of smoking occurred for the first 5 weeks followed by 2 weeks of cessation. The second phase was an 8-week follow-up interval where subjects were assigned to one of four groups: (1) no contact, (2) self-monitoring and mailed-in results, (3) telephone contact every two weeks and (4) telephone contact and self-monitoring. At the end of Phase 2 all subjects attended one group meeting to hand in questionnaires. Phase 3 was a longer follow-up interval with no contact, taking between 3 and 5.5 months.

Subjects who endorsed a high value on health smoked significantly less (16.9 cpd) than low health value (28.9 cpd). High health value subjects maintained lowered smoking rates. Low health value subjects often returned to baseline smoking levels. Internal HLC subjects achieved greater reductions than external HLC subjects at all measurement periods. The results from this study support the theory that situation-specific measures of expectancies and values were useful in the prediction of situation-specific behaviors. The authors discussed the implications of these findings and ways to change health values and locus of control beliefs.

81.   Lando, H. A., & McCullough, J. A. (1978). Clinical application of a broad-spectrum behavioral approach to chronic smokers. Journal of Consulting and Clinical Psychology, 46(6), 1583-1585.

The study was a replication of Lando's (1977) findings with the addition of a maintained reduction by non-abstinent smokers. Seventeen subjects had a mean age of 35.7 years and an average smoking history of 28.7 cpd for 17.3 years. All subjects received six aversion treatment sessions over one week. Subjects were told to smoke as much as possible, followed by abstinence. Seven maintenance sessions had group discussions, contract signing and self-reward/punishment for acceptance/breach of contract. Subjects who failed abstinence were reorientated toward maintained reductions with contracts and self-reward/punishment. Twelve of the 16 remained abstinent at 4- and 6-month follow-up. Two subjects were assigned to maintained reductions. Both subjects successfully maintained reductions substantially lower than baseline. The authors achieved a large successful abstinence rate. Caution was required about interpretation, however, due to the small sample size and due to loosely implemented "maintained reduction" procedures.

82.   Schinke, S. P., Blythe, B. J., & Doueck, H. J. (1978). Reducing cigarette smoking: Evaluation of a multifaceted interventive program. Behavioral Engineering, 4 (4), 107-112.

The clinical efficacy of a multifaceted intervention package of smoking reduction techniques was investigated. Eight subjects who averaged 34.16 years, with a mean smoking history of 34 cpd for 18 years expressed interest in reduced cigarette consumption. Six subjects were assigned to the experimental condition and two to a no-intervention control condition. All subjects used a wrist counter to record cigarette urges. They recorded urges to smoke and cigarettes smoked on a monitoring sheet. Monitoring occurred for the first 8 weeks. Weekly records were kept at 1-, 3- and 6-month follow-up. The experimental condition consisted of eight, 90 minute group sessions. Individual stimulus conditions and environmental cues for smoking were identified and discussed. Each subject using the previous week's data constructed a graph of daily urges and cigarettes smoked. Changes in stimulus conditions or smoking behavior were given special attention. Rapid smoking or handling of cigarette litter and covert sensitization (for subjects in poor health) was administered for two sessions. Relaxation techniques and refusal behavior rehearsals were presented and practiced. Experimental subjects reported a reduction in post-treatment urges and number of cigarettes smoked, compared to baseline. Follow-up data at 1-, 3- and 6-months post-treatment showed that experimental subjects continued to experience less urges. They also smoked fewer cigarettes than control subjects.

These results supported the efficacy of a multifaceted intervention package for reduced cigarette smoking.

83.   Colletti, G., & Kopel, S. A. (1979). Maintaining behavior change: An investigation of three maintenance strategies and the relationship of self-attribution to the long-term reduction of cigarette smoking. Journal of Consulting and Clinical Psychology, 47(3), 614-617.

Forty-two subjects gave an average age of 37.68 years and mean smoking history of 32.11 cpd for 20.66 years. All subjects attended an identical 4-week treatment stage of two, 1-hour sessions a week with six to nine people in a group. The treatment included: daily self-monitoring and charting the weekly smoking rates, a review of individual smoking patterns, suggestions of stimulus control techniques for each subject and discussion of smoking-related health hazards. After treatment, subjects were randomly assigned to either Modeling (M) where subjects acted as models for new subjects about to receive treatment, Participant Observing (PO) a control group for M where subjects were in a group but not specifically encouraged to serve as models, or self-monitoring (SM) with minimal phone contact only. All groups maintained significant smoking reductions at 1 year with an average of 46% of baseline. The results suggested that maintenance procedures were effective but the particular strategy used was less important. The authors concluded that SM was the best approach, due to equivalent success rates and low cost. The second group to receive treatment (the observers for the M and PO groups) consisted of 32 subjects, and showed similar reductions from baseline to the groups they observed (either M or PO).

84.   Merbaum, M., Avimier, R., & Goldberg, J. (1979). The relationship between aversion, group training and vomiting in the reduction of smoking behavior. Addictive Behaviors, 4(3), 279-285.

The aim of the study was to compare the efficacy of two levels of induced aversion (single level and combined). It was predicted that: strong aversion plus group contact would be more successful than strong aversion alone, strong aversion would be more successful than mild aversion and that more vomiting during aversion training would result in less smoking at follow-up. Fifty-two volunteer subjects were recruited from a community in Israel. Subjects gave a mean age of 34.32 years and mean smoking history of 28.25 cpd for 13.5 years. Group 1 (strong aversion) received satiation plus covert sensitization for 1.5 hours on six consecutive days. Group 2 (strong aversion plus self-control) received the same treatment as group 1, followed by self-control training in a group setting for 1½ hours a week for six consecutive weeks. Group 3, (strong aversion plus temptation control) received the same treatment as group 1 followed by temptation control training in a group setting for 1½ hours a week for 6 consecutive weeks. Group 4 (mild aversion) received satiation for 1½ hours on six consecutive days. Frequency of vomiting episodes was recorded for each group. Follow-up assessments occurred at two and six months.

Results showed 69% abstinence at the end of the aversive treatment week. Group 1 and 2 were superior to the other groups in abstinence rates at 6-month follow-up. The advantages of a treatment package over aversive treatment were not demonstrated. Significant reductions of baseline smoking by non-abstainers were not achieved. The results showed that unless abstinence was achieved, most subjects returned to initial baseline smoking levels. Results also suggested that vomiting during treatment might be related to reduced cigarette consumption post-treatment.

85.   Colletti, G., & Stern, L. (1980). Two year follow up of a non-aversive treatment for cigarette smoking. Journal of Consulting and Clinical Psychology, 48 (2), 292-293.

A 2-year follow-up was reported for 72 of 74 subjects involved in a smoking reduction program. After non-aversive treatment (involving self-monitoring, stimulus control and discussion) subjects were assigned to one of three maintenance strategies: Modeling (M) in which previous subjects served as models for new subjects about to receive treatment; participant observing (PO) where subjects were given support for participation but not specifically encouraged to serve as models (a control for M group); and self-monitoring (SM) where subjects continued self-monitoring and had contact with the therapist by phone only. Smoking rates were collected by phone or post and estimated over a 3-day period. At 2-year follow-up, mean smoking rate was 51.23% of baseline and a 24% abstinence rate from the original sample was observed. Fifty-six percent maintained abstinence from 1-year follow-up. No significant relapse had occurred from 1 to 2 year follow-ups, and all 3 groups had maintained meaningful reductions from baseline. The SM group compared to the M observed superior maintenance of smoking reductions and PO groups. The lower cost of SM as a maintenance strategy (with the less time and intensity involved) were arguments for its efficacy. The 2-year outcomes for the 32 newcomer subjects who had observed either the M or PO group were parallel to the group observed, suggesting replicability of results. Satisfaction with the program and self-labeling as a non-smoker at 1-year follow-up was correlated with favourable 2-year outcome. It was suggested that these variables might be predictors of favorable long-term outcome.

86.   Beaver, C., Brown, R. A., & Lichtenstein, E. (1981). Effects of monitored nicotine fading and anxiety management training on smoking reduction. Addictive Behaviors, 6(4), 301-305.

The study examined the effect of anxiety management on nicotine fading treatment for smoking reduction. It was predicted that anxiety management would be more helpful for subjects high in trait anxiety. Twenty-six subjects with a mean age of 30.1 years and a mean 13.1 smoking years completed the study. Subjects were assigned to high and low anxiety groups based on a median split of Trait Anxiety Inventory scores. Subjects were then randomly assigned to nicotine fading (NF) treatment or nicotine fading plus anxiety management (NF+AM). Subjects were given treatment in small groups, once a week for six weeks. NF group followed the general procedure for nicotine fading and self-monitoring. Group support was emphasized and a tip sheet with alternative non-smoking behaviors was distributed. NF+AM received NF for the first 3 sessions and AM. This had relaxation training and covert rehearsal during the last 3 sessions. Follow-up assessment occurred at 1-week, 1-, 3-, and 6-months. Smoking rates showed the characteristic sharp relapse effect during the first 3 months post-treatment. The effect was less but still significant for nicotine intake. Subject who received AM did worse than NF alone. The poorest results were obtained for subjects of high anxiety. Of the 21 subjects still smoking at 6-month follow-up, 18 had reduced nicotine content relative to baseline with a median reduction of 0.6 mg. Results also showed that subjects did not increase rate of smoking to compensate for reduced nicotine content.

87.   Lando, H. A. (1981). Effects of preparation, experimenter contact, and a maintained reduction alternative on a broad-spectrum program for eliminating smoking. Addictive Behaviors, 6 (2), 123-133.

The study compared three variables, treatment stages (2 vs. 3 stage program), experimenter contact (intensive vs. minimal), and tracking (goal of abstinence vs. maintained reductions for non-abstinence). Ninety-nine subjects had a mean age of 37.5 years and a mean smoking history of 32.3 cpd for 19.0 years. Baseline smoking was determined, and then treatment occurred in groups of 7-12 subjects. The three-stage treatment consisted of preparation (introducing stimulus control and fear appeal), aversion (continuous laboratory smoking with abstinence between sessions, "unlearning" by smoking at least twice the usual rate in the lead up to a cessation date) and maintenance (follow-up sessions for discussion and contract signing and booster sessions following relapse).   The two-stage program omitted the preparation stage.   Minimal Contact group was taught self-administration of treatments in three sessions compared to the 15- and 13-sessions for intensive contact.   Tracking was made available randomly to half the subjects who had relapsed and failed. Booster sessions consisted of stimulus control and contracts that limited smoking to a level not less than 10 cpd, but not more than 50% of baseline.

A 58% abstinence rate at 6 months and 46% at 12 months for the 2-stage program replicated previous success. Superiority over the 3-stage program was demonstrated.   Two-stage subjects performed better under intensive contact while 3-stage subjects performed better with minimal contact.   Excessive information and group cohesiveness may explain these effects.   Disappointing tracking manipulation results were reported and discussed.   It was suggested that tracking procedures might be inappropriate as a post hoc alternative to an abstinence program.   Controlled smoking procedures (with reduced risk rather than a goal of abstinence) were suggested as an alternative.

88.   Poole, A. D., Sanson-Fisher, R. W., & German, G. A. (1981). The rapid-smoking technique: Therapeutic effectiveness. Behaviour Research and Therapy, 19 (5), 389-397.

Seventy-five subjects participated after passing a medical-examination. They had a mean age of 32.2 years and mean smoking history of 28.4 cpd for 14.4 years.   At an initial session a refundable deposit was collected and Eysenck Personality Inventory, Locus of Control scale, smoking history, Motivation to stop smoking and Expectation of success questionnaires were completed.   Smoking behavior for the next seven days was recorded. Subjects in group 1-3 met in groups of three or four people. Subjects in group 4 were treated individually. Group 1 were given a rapid smoking procedure. They were encouraged to complete 3 trials per session for a minimum of 6 sessions or a maximum of 12 sessions, or until abstinence was maintained between sessions. Group 2 received rapid smoking and relaxation. Two sessions were devoted to individual smoking behavior analysis, training in self-control and relaxation procedures. Group 3 received the same procedures as group 2 but also included contingency contracting to reinforce abstinence. Group 4 received rapid smoking like group 1, individually for the initial session. This was followed by 3 sessions in

6 days, repeated until the subject and the 'significant other' agreed on abstinence between sessions. During the maintenance period of 9 weeks, abstinence was checked and booster sessions held when required.

The study reported 64% abstinence after treatment with 21% at 12 months. Excluding abstainers, 34% reduction of baseline cigarette consumption at post-treatment relapsed to 82% of baseline at 12-month follow-up. There were no major differences in abstinence or reduction rates between groups. Self-control, relaxation and contingency contracts did not improve results in a rapid smoking program. These results were compared to other studies of rapid smoking. Abstinence and reduction effectiveness as a treatment for smoking was discussed.

89.   Nicki, R. M., Remington, R. E., & MacDonald, G. A. (1984). Self-efficacy, nicotine-fading/self-monitoring and cigarette-smoking behavior. Behaviour Research and Therapy, 22 (5), 477-485.

This study was a replication and extension of Foxx & Brown's (1979) nicotine fading self-monitoring (NFSM) procedure for smoking abstinence or control. This included an analysis of the effects of self-instruction (SI) training and self-efficacy (SE) training. Forty-five subjects completed treatment. Eight subjects were a control group, with an average smoking history of one pack of cigarettes a day containing at least 0.8 mg of nicotine for an average of 10 years. The control group was contacted for an estimate of smoking behavior both initially and at 12-month follow-up. Group 1 received NFSM, group 2 received NFSM and SI, group 3 received NFSM and SE, and group 4 received NFSM and both SI and SE. NFSM involved the sequential weekly reductions of nicotine content by changing brand of cigarettes smoked over 3 weeks to a point of abstinence. The daily total nicotine intake was plotted on a graph. SI training involved cognitive restructuring in cigarette smoking situations involving a four-stage format of preparation, confronting, coping and reinforcing. SE training involved smoking cessation in more situations, starting with the easiest and progressing to the most difficult.

A significant reduction for all treatments in both number of cigarettes smoked per week (73% from baseline) and mean nicotine intake (97% of baseline) occurred by post-treatment follow-up. The reductions remained fairly stable between 5-month and 12-month follow-up. There was 34% reduction from baseline in mean number and 71% reduction from baseline in mean nicotine intake. SI and /or SE training produced no increase in treatment effectiveness for reduction, but SE training did seem to aid in cessation. The importance of self-efficacy in the treatment of smoking was discussed.

90.   Suedfeld, P., & Baker-Brown, G. (1986). Restricted Environmental Stimulation Therapy and aversive conditioning in smoking cessation: Active and placebo effects. Behavior Research and Therapy, 24 (4), 421-428.

A subtractive expectancy placebo technique was used to investigate the active and placebo effects in Restricted Environment Stimulation Therapy (REST) and aversive conditioning. Seventy-four subjects gave a mean age of 35 years, and baseline smoking of 34 cpd for 19 years. Group 1 received aversive conditioning in the form of imagined scenes and one day of satiation smoking. Subjects were told they should smoke twice the usual cigarette consumption. Group 2 received the same treatment as group 1 followed by REST for 24 hours. REST involved 24 hours in a completely dark sound-reducing room with water and liquid diet food available through a plastic tube near a pillow on a bed. Group 3 received the same treatment as group 2 but REST was described as a recuperation period in a relaxation room. Subjects were told that it was not part of the treatment. Group 4 received the same treatment as group 2 but the aversive conditioning satiation smoking was a demonstration procedure. Subjects were told that it was not part of the treatment. Follow-ups occurred at 3-, 6-, 9-, and 12-months post-treatment. Group 2 reported the largest reduction at 1-year follow-up (55%) with all the other groups about 40%. The combined treatments were more effective than aversive conditioning alone. The results supported the hypothesis that subjects treated with REST were less likely to relapse once they had quit smoking. Subjects that did not quit showed success in controlled smoking.

91.   Reynolds, R. V. C., Tobin, D. L., Creer, T. L., Wigal, J. K., & Wagner, M. D. (1987). A method for studying controlled substance use: A preliminary investigation. Addictive Behaviors, 12, 53-62.

The study examined relapse after treatment in a smoking reduction program using a set of cognitive, smoking history, and reduction motivation variables. Twenty-two subjects attended more than half the eight treatment sessions, and gave an average age of 37.1 years, and average smoking history of 25.7 cpd for 20 years. All subjects completed a questionnaire pre-treatment about demographics, smoking history, and motivation to quit smoking. A post-treatment questionnaire included satisfaction with the program, expectancy to maintain gains, degree of self-labeling as a non-smoker, maintenance motivation, self-efficacy scale, smokers' locus of control scale and the self-consciousness scale. Treatment was a controlled smoking self-management program in eight 1-hour group sessions over four weeks. The program included self-analysis of individual smoking habits, stimulus control procedures, self-reinforcement of behaviors incompatible with smoking, health-risk information, progressive muscle relaxation, and group support. Reduction goals were set at each session with abstinence encouraged, but a 50% reduction from baseline acceptable as a post-treatment reduction goal.

Post-treatment smoking was significantly lower than pre-treatment smoking. Slight relapse was reported at 3-month follow-up. Motivation to reduce smoking accounted for more variance in post-treatment smoking than any of the smoking history variables. Degree of self-labeling as a non-smoker and internal smokers' locus of control accounted for a significant amount of variance (50.8%) of smoking at 3-month follow-up. Limitations of the study and directions for future research were suggested.

92.   Wheeler, R. J. (1988). Effects of a community-wide smoking cessation program. Social Science and Medicine, 27(12), 1387-1392.

A telephone survey was used to determine the effect of a low cost community-wide smoking cessation campaign. This involved a 20-day self-conducted "freedom from smoking" program with television and radio coverage. A total of 42,500 manuals were distributed amongst an estimated 690,000 smokers in the target area. Seventy-three percent of the people (30,940) who received the manual started the program. The average age of the participants was 42.2 years, the average age on onset was 17.2 years and the mean years smoking was 22.3. The survey reported that 80% of participants had tried to quit previously, with 30% abstinent for 6 months or more. The mean number of cigarettes smoked each day was 29.9 of 0.8-mg nicotine content.

Generalizing data from the telephone survey to the overall population suggested that 5,300 stopped smoking; 26,500 reduced their smoking from an average of 33 to 17.9 cpd. Published information about the cost of smoking suggested this community-based program saved about 14 million dollars, ranging from health care costs to cigarette savings for the target population. Only 37% of participants used the manual for the 20-day program. Most participants used it less than six times. An aid (most commonly food or candy) was used by 43% of participants to assist smoking cessation. Social support was reported as important to assist smoking cessation, with non-smokers more helpful than smokers. Participants who made the largest reductions were found to have smoked more at baseline, and those who success-fully quit tended to stop abruptly early in the program. The author expressed hope the results would encourage more media-based programs for communities.

93.   Graybar, S. R., Antonuccio, D. O., Boutilier, L. R., & Varble, D. L. (1989). Psychological reactance as a factor affecting patient compliance to physician advice. Scandinavian Journal of Behaviour Therapy, 18(1), 43-51.

The purpose of the study was to examine the relationship between patient reactance and physician advice to quit smoking. The 3 independent variables were reactance, tone and amount of physician advice. It was hypothesized that the use of negative advice would produce more arousal of reactance and less compliance to quit smoking than positive advice; and subjects high in reactance, high amounts of physician advice would produce less compliance than low amounts of advice. One hundred and four subjects met the study criteria and completed initial measures. Subjects averaged 59.9 years of age, 21.7 cpd and 11.6 years of education and were randomly assigned to one of five treatment groups. Subjects completed a smoking questionnaire and a Therapeutic Reactance questionnaire prior to consultation with a physician who gave either a low amount (1-2 minutes) of quit advice in a positive tone (group 1), low amount in a negative tone (group 2), high amount (5 minutes) in a positive tone (group 3), or high amount in a negative tone (group 4). The control group (group 5) completed all questionnaires, was given a quit pamphlet but did not discuss quitting with their physician. Follow-up questionnaires were sent to subjects one month after initial contact. Post-treatment data were obtained for 95 subjects and revealed nine abstinent. Eight subjects signed up for a smoking cessation program. Data showed a significant relationship between the amount of advice and behavioral reactance. This indicated subjects low in behavioral reactance responded better to high amounts of advice. It was also found that subjects high in behavioral reactance achieved the greatest reductions when given low amounts of negatively toned advice. Theoretical and practical implications were discussed.

94.   Lee, C. (1991). Evaluation of a self-help smoking cessation program. Behaviour Change, 8 (2), 87-93.

Forty-one subjects had a mean age of 40 years, mean smoking history of 27 cpd for 22 years. Thirty-four subjects had an average of 2 previous unsuccessful attempts at quitting. All subjects received a smoking cessation booklet with four chapters. Subjects were told to finish all activities in each chapter before starting the next. Chapter 1 involved a range of preparatory activities including self-monitoring (to measure baseline), information, individual cues, and relaxation techniques. Chapter 2 was the 'stopping' phase where a date was set to halve the baseline smoking rate and complete cessation aimed for 3 days later. Contracting, behavioral rehearsal for high-risk situations and relapse training were included. Chapter 3 was the initial maintenance stage, which mainly consisted of repetition and development of activities in earlier sections. Self-monitoring, behavioral rehearsal and relapse training were revised with supplementary advice on diet and health. Chapter 4 was a subsequent maintenance stage and was again largely a repetition of earlier material with an additional long-term contract completion. Participants completed several questionnaires including self-efficacy and the Multidimensional Health Locus of Control Scale. Subjects were contacted by telephone at 2- and 4-weeks, 3-, 6- and 12-months follow-up, and reports of smoking cessation were checked with a saliva sample.

A significant reduction in smoking rate was reported between baseline, 2 and 4 week assessments (26.7, 15.6, 9.3 cpd respectively). Ten subjects reported abstinence at their last contact. Several subjects became controlled smokers, and reduced their smoking rate to 2 or 3 cpd, maintained for several months with no reported intentions to change. The authors commented that controlled smoking was not an intentional outcome of the study. Reduced health risks in chronic heavy smokers may be possible.

95.   Kumari, V., Kaushik, S. S., & Singh, R. (1993). Experimental analysis and modification of smoking behaviour through behavioural techniques. Indian Journal of Clinical Psychology, 20(1), 43-49.

The study was designed to evaluate the effects of a behavioral package to control smoking via an experimental design. During an initial interview subjects were selected who had smoked 10-20 cpd for more than 5 years and who had started smoking mostly for the reason of company. The 4 subjects completed several questionnaires. After the exclusion of 2 subjects, the remaining subjects were matched on their questionnaire answers. The therapist and subject decided on a smoking reduction target that was no less than 90% reduction from baseline. Behavior analysis was performed in each phase of the study.

The case history of each subject was presented with the reduction target. Subjects recorded frequency of smoking and intensity of urges during the assigned baseline period. A 3 week self-control quit smoking program followed, which involved changing cigarette brand, not smoking for 1 hour before breakfast or going to sleep, brushing teeth, flossing, gargling with diluted hydrogen peroxide, and practice of relaxation techniques. This routine was introduced instead of post-meal smoking and smoking all day between meals. Follow-up occurred at 1 and 9 months. One subject achieved his goal of abstinence and maintained it at the 9 month follow-up. The other subject did not achieve his goal of 90% reduction but did achieve a substantial reduction. He was still smoking less at the 9 month follow-up. The progress and problems for each subject was discussed. It was concluded that individual factors of participants should be taken into consideration when preparing a behavioral package for the modification of smoking.

4

CHARACTERISTICS AND PROCESS

96.   Russell, M. A. H., Wilson, C., Cole, P. V., Idle, M., & Feyerabend, C. (1973). Comparison of increases in carboxyhaemoglobin after smoking "extra-mild" and "non-mild" cigarettes. Lancet, 2, 687-690.

Changes in carboxyhaemoglobin (COHb) levels as a result of changing to "extra mild" and "non mild" cigarettes were analysed to assess the effect of carbon monoxide (CO) changes in tobacco smoke and reducing the harmfulness of cigarettes. Twenty-two smokers were assigned to one of two groups. Group 1 smoked standard size cigarettes with half smoking extra mild (A) before non mild (B) and other half smoking B then A. Group 2 smoked small size cigarettes, again with half smoking extra mild (C) followed by non mild (D) and the other half smoking D than C. Venous blood samples were collected before and after two laboratory smoked cigarettes. Subjects were instructed to smoke ten puffs for standard size cigarettes and seven puffs for small size cigarettes with 40 seconds between each puff and 20 minutes between each cigarette. The mean increase in COHb level after smoking a single B cigarette was 1.45%. The mean COHb increase after smoking a single D cigarette was 1.09%. The mean COHb increase after smoking a single A cigarette was 0.64%. The mean COHb increase after smoking a single C cigarette was 0.75%. The CO absorption from the standard size mild cigarette was less than half the amount absorbed from the non-mild cigarette. It is observed that the low CO brand also had a low tar and nicotine yield. The health implications of variations in CO yield of cigarettes are discussed as equally important to those of tar and nicotine yield.

97.   Turner, J. A., Sillett, R. W., & Ball, K. P. (1974). Some effects of changing to low-tar and low-nicotine cigarettes. Lancet, 2, 737-739.

Cigarette consumption, blood carboxyhaemoglobin (COHb) levels and smoking patterns were analysed in 10 subjects to study the effect of changing to low tar and low nicotine cigarettes. The subjects averaged 32 years with a mean consumption of 28 cpd containing 16-20 mg of tar and 1.0-1.3 mg nicotine. The tar and nicotine yields of the baseline cigarettes were classified as medium (only one subject smoked low yields at baseline). Subjects smoked medium strength cigarettes (19-20 mg tar, 1.4 mg nicotine) during week 1, low strength cigarettes (12 mg tar, 0.8 mg nicotine) during week 2 and very low strength cigarettes (4 mg tar and <0.3 mg nicotine) during week 3. Venous blood samples were taken at the end of at least 5 days of each smoking period. Subjects self-monitored smoking behavior, gave a satisfaction rating of each brand smoked, and some butts were collected and analysed for length of tobacco unsmoked and nicotine content.

Cigarette consumption increased significantly during the low and very low periods compared to the medium period. The mean COHb for the medium period was 6.34%, 6.25% for the low period and a significant drop to 3.80% for the very low period. More complete smoking of the low and very low brands were shown by shorter butt length and changes in filter nicotine content, indicating that smoking may be related to nicotine intake. However, changes in consumption did not show a complete picture for nicotine compensation. The reduction in COHb levels did not correlate with the expected CO dose predicted. A close correlation between the expected CO dose predicted, and the actual CO dose (from the change in smoking pattern) was found. It is concluded that very low tar and nicotine cigarettes may reduce the hazards of smoking by reducing the CO and nicotine doses.

98.   Joyce, A. M., O'Rourke, T. W., & O'Rourke, D. M. (1976). Assessment of the perceived impact of taxation upon smoking behavior: Implications for health education. Journal of Drug Education, 6(3), 231-240.

The perceived impact on smoking behavior of increased taxation on cigarettes was analysed. A brief survey with the primary emphasis on the perceived impact of cigarette taxation was completed by 259 students. The sample contained 74% of students under the age of 20 years. Results indicated equivalent numbers favoured the tax increase as were opposed to the tax increase, and further analysis indicated that non-smokers and ex-smokers favoured the tax increase more than smokers. Most smokers indicated that they would stop or cut-down smoking if the tax increase was initiated. All subjects indicated they thought smoking reductions would occur as a result of the tax increases. All subjects also indicated that the higher the tax increase, the larger the reduction or cessation incidence. The limitations, including a college student sample with generalisation problems, and analysis of perceived reactions to the proposed situation, were acknowledged by the author.

99.   Perri, M. G., Richards, C. S., & Schultheis, K. R. (1977). Behavioral self-control and smoking reduction: A study of self-initiated attempts to reduce smoking. Behavior Therapy, 8(3), 360-365.

The procedures used to self-control smoking behavior were investigated using a structured interview procedure given to people who successfully or unsuccessfully reduced smoking. Twenty four successful and 24 unsuccessful subjects were selected from an undergraduate sample of students who had a serious smoking problem and had made a concerted effort to reduce or quit smoking. Successful subjects were classified as those who decreased the number of cigarettes smoked per day by 50% or more, maintained for at least 4 months and were satisfied with their reduced smoking rate. The interview collected information such as smoking history, methods used to reduce smoking, the implementation and effects of the methods used and current smoking status. Successful subjects rated themselves as more motivated to personal change, used a greater number of techniques more frequently, consistently and longer than unsuccessful subjects. Successful self-controllers also rated their techniques as more practical and used positive feedback, self-reinforcement techniques and problem solving procedures than did unsuccessful subjects. Limitations and benefits of the study are discussed.

100.   Blittner, M., & Goldberg, J. (1978). Cognitive self-control factors in the reduction of smoking behavior. Behavior Therapy, 9, 553-561.

Non-specific factors such as motivation, beliefs, and expectations are described as influential variables of behavior modification. It has been suggested that these variables could account for the apparent similarity of results in most therapy programs including modification of smoking behavior. It was expected that a therapeutic approach which emphasized the cognitive stage that establishes and reinforces a self-control belief system and included a training stage in specific self-control procedures would be more effective in maintaining a reduction in smoking than a treatment approach concerned only with stimulus control training. Fifty-four Israeli subjects from 2 kibbutzim were placed in three groups matched on age and smoking history (28 cpd for 16 years). In addition, subject motivation to stop smoking and expectancy of success were equivalent for each group. The first group was told they had shown from a battery of projective tests that they had strong willpower and the ability to control and change their behavior. The second group were told they were selected at random for treatment in stimulus discrimination training which was also given to the first group. The third group served as a control group who received no treatment and were given no feedback on test performance.

During the follow-up period the Yom Kippur War began and due to this unpredicted stressful situation, the entire process was replicated on the same subjects following the initial 6 month follow-up. Data obtained at the initial 6-month follow-up was also used as baseline data for the second treatment phase. Significant differences were found between each groups at post-treatment, 3.5 month and 6 month follow-up. A large relapse following the first treatment is attributed to the stress of the war, but group 1 reduced cigarette smoking to 30% of baseline and group 2 to 70% of baseline by the second treatment 3 month follow-up. It is concluded that this study supports the addition of a cognitive support system which reinforces the idea of inner control to the smoking treatment program to enhance reduction.

101.   Castelli, W. P., Garrison, R. J., Dawber, T. R., McNamara, P. M., Feinleib, M., & Kannel, W. B. (1981). The filter cigarette and Coronary Heart Disease: The Framingham study. Lancet, 109-113.

It was hypothesised that those who smoke filter cigarettes are less likely to get clinical manifestations of Coronary Heart Disease (CHD) than those who smoke non-filter cigarettes. The Framingham Heart Study Cohort participants underwent physical examinations biannually since 1948. Data about cigarette filter use was collected for the first time in Examination 7 (E7), and then again in Examination 12 (E12). Data from E7 formed the baseline for comparisons. Only those subjects who formed the baseline were considered in data presented for the 1st or 12th examinations, or other follow-ups. One thousand six hundred and five men and 2132 women aged 41-74 were involved in E7. It was observed that only the youngest women smoked cigarettes therefore the data for women was omitted. Fifty-eight percent of the cigarette smoking men under the age of 55 used filters. These men had slightly less history in smoking than non-filter cigarette smokers and it was found that they did not have lower CHD incidence rates than non-filter smokers. This result remained unchanged even after adjustments were made for differences in age, systolic blood pressure, and serum cholesterol. The authors conclude that evidence was not provided in the Framingham Study to support the promise of the filter philosophy; that toxins which cause degradation of lung function, cancer, and CHD are removed, and therefore the effectiveness for the safer cigarette is questionable.

102.   Hughes, J. R., Epstein, L. H., Andrasik, F., Neff, D. F., & Thompson, D. S. (1982). Smoking and carbon monoxide levels during pregnancy. Addictive Behaviors, 7(3), 271-276.

The study was aimed to evaluate the validity of carbon monoxide (CO) as a measure of smoking status during pregnancy and to describe smoking behavior during pregnancy. At a women's' hospital 167 pregnant women completed self-reports, medical and CO data. Most subjects (72%) were less than 25 years of age, in their third trimester (61%), had finished high school (71%), were unemployed (63%), were unmarried (56%), and were in a moderate to low socioeconomic group. A comparison of smoking self-reports and CO analysis found agreement of smoking status in 88% of cases and the authors suggest that breath CO is a valid objective measure of smoking status in pregnant as well as non-pregnant women. Of the women who smoked at the beginning of their pregnancy, 66% reported abstinence or reductions by the time of the survey. Most of these quit or reduced in their first trimester, stating pregnancy related reasons but the factors responsible were not determined. The authors suggest treatment programs for smoking during pregnancy should be aimed at women early in their pregnancy and intervention should occur during prenatal outpatient visits due to poor attendance at smoking clinics.

103.   Russell, M. A. H., Sutton, S. R., Feyerabend, C., & Vesey, C. J. (1982). Long-term switching to low-tar low-nicotine cigarettes. British Journal of Addiction, 77, 145-158.

The study reported the changes in blood nicotine, cotinine, carboxy-haemoglobin (COHb) and thiocyanate (SCN) levels in 12 smokers before and after switching to a low-tar, low-nicotine cigarette for 10 weeks. The subjects averaged 37.3 years with a mean cigarette consumption of 37.9 cpd containing 17.4 mg tar, 1.33 mg nicotine, 17.0 mg carbon monoxide (CO), and averaging 76.2 mm in length. At each session cigarette consumption for the day was recorded, a cigarette was smoked on a puff analyser, venous blood samples were taken at various times, COHb was analysed and plasma nicotine measured. Nicotine content of cigarette butts smoked that day were measured and ratings of satisfaction and taste were recorded.

There was no significant change in cigarette consumption on switching from usual brands to low-tar cigarettes. The mouth level intake of nicotine was significantly reduced after switching to the low yield cigarettes, and plasma nicotine levels reduced substantially. Plasma cotinine is a main metabolite of nicotine and reflects the nicotine intake from all cigarettes smoked during the day. Plasma cotinine analysis was performed in a limited number of samples and supported the plasma nicotine data showing an identical and significant reduction of 30% at eight and ten weeks after switching to low-yield cigarettes. No significant changes in COHb or plasma SCN were recorded. No significant changes in puff volume, total volume puffed, puff rate and time taken to smoke the cigarette were observed. In the long term the low-yield cigarettes were preferred to the usual brand and intentions of permanent changes were reported. The degree of compensation on switching to low-yield cigarettes was only partial and did not significantly alter after 8-10 weeks. It was concluded that although compensation can occur by increasing inhalation, heavy smokers with difficulty in abstinence could benefit by switching to low-yield cigarettes.

104.   Rosen, T. J., & Shipley, R. H. (1983). A stage analysis of self-initiated smoking reductions. Addictive Behaviors, 8(3), 263-272.

The value of analysing smoking cessation in three stages, decision, initial control, and maintenance, was investigated. Smokers who received a free breath carbon monoxide measure at a "Health Fair" were invited to participate in a study of smoking behavior, and analysis was performed on 61 subjects in the pre-test sample, 51 in the follow-up sample (between 1-2 months after initial contact) and 23 in the "tried to reduce" sample. Questionnaires included background information, predictor measures of self-esteem, Health Locus of Control, desire to stop and self-efficacy. Questionnaires were given at pre-test and follow-up. The follow-up questionnaire allowed calculation of a relapse score from information about efforts made to reduce or stop smoking and the lowest reported cigarette consumption. The 51 subjects at follow-up smoked an average of 85.5% of baseline. Of the 23 subjects who tried to reduce, the greatest reduction from baseline was 31.7% and the mean relapse was to 76.8% of baseline. The 'tried to reduce' criterion was identified with the decision stage, the lowest percent of baseline with initial control stage, and relapse criterion with the maintenance stage. Self-esteem was the variable related to Lowest Percent of Baseline and no evidence was found to link emotional factors with relapse. It was found that subjects with high desire to stop and internal Health Locus of Control tended to resist relapse. It is concluded that differences among stages highlight the importance of smoking treatment programs which change over time to best match the smokers needs.

105.   Sjoberg, L. (1983). Value change and relapse following a decision to quit or reduce smoking. Scandinavian Journal of Psychology, 24 (2), 137-148.

The validity of the Value Model and the Action Model in a number of smokers during an attempt to quit or reduce smoking was investigated. The Value Model is concerned with the change of values over time while the Action Model suggests the choice options are differentiated as a function of commitment to action. Exploratory data on relevant experience and techniques used in fighting temptations were also analysed. Twenty-three subjects had an average age of 27.3 years and mean smoking history of 23 cpd for 10.7 years, and were willing to quit (n=12) or reduce smoking to 50% (n=11) for one week. Questionnaires were completed each day for seven days and contained background data, attitude, rating selected events and states, probability of success or failure and importance ratings, activities, mood at times of failures, experience ratings (of events and states) and perceived persistence.

The Value Model was not supported by the data. Both alternatives 'smoke' and 'not smoke' were negative, with the first being more negative, suggesting the possibility that the two negative options generate an avoidance-avoidance conflict. Failure could not be predicted from experience ratings although some variation, especially in somatic value variables could be seen. The Action Model was more successful in accounting for the time changes as subjects became more distinct and clear in their thinking of the two choice options, and committed to one. However, neither approaches were successful in accounting for relapses. Action was hard to predict from beliefs and values and may be more successfully accounted for by desires and emotional states.

106.   Alderson, M. R., Lee, P. N., & Wang, R. (1985). Risks of lung cancer, chronic bronchitis, ischaemic heart disease, and stroke in relation to type of cigarette smoked. Journal of Epidemiology and Community Health. 39, 286-293.

A case control study of hospital inpatients examined the risk of lung cancer, chronic bronchitis, ischaemic heart disease and stroke with type of cigarette smoked. Twelve thousand, six hundred and ninety-three interviews of patients aged 35-74 recorded information on current smoking status, detailed smoking history, initial diagnosis and discharge diagnosis. In both sexes cigarette smoking was highly significantly associated with lung cancer, chronic bronchitis, and in the 35-54 age group ischaemic heart disease. It was not significantly related to ischaemic heart disease or stroke in older patients. Risks of lung cancer and chronic bronchitis were higher (but not significantly) in handrolled rather than manufactured cigarette smokers. Smoking was more strongly associated with squamous and small cell lung cancer than other types of lung cancer. Risk of lung cancer was significantly decreased among long term ex-smokers, but not clearly related to time of switching from plain to filter cigarettes. The lowest tar group (brand of cigarette smoked 10 years before admission) generally had the lowest risk. Chronic bronchitis in males significantly showed twice the risk for smokers of brands with tar yields 29+ mg compared to smokers of brands with 17-22 mg of tar. The validity of data collection is discussed and it is concluded that this study is compatible with others in suggesting that risk of lung cancer and chronic bronchitis is probably reduced by switching from plain to filter cigarettes.

107.   Devins, G. M., & Edwards, P. J. (1988). Self-efficacy and smoking reduction in Chronic Obstructive Pulmonary Disease. Behaviour Research and Therapy, 26 (2), 127-135.

It is reported that Chronic Obstructive Pulmonary Disease (COPD) patients who stop or reduce smoking can reverse or partially reverse the deterioration in lung function and difficulty in breathing to that of normal aging. Two specific cognitions, efficacy and outcome expectation in Banduras Social Cognitive Theory (SCT) have been hypothesised to play key roles in achieving behavioral changes like smoking reduction. This study hypothesised that self-efficacy would be the only SCT variable to be a significant predictor of smoking reduction or cessation. It was further hypothesised that interactions of self-efficacy with repertoire, motivation, and outcome expectancies would be related to reduced smoking but the main effects of each upon smoking behavior would be non significant. Forty-five diagnosed COPD patients with a mean age of 55.6 years and a mean smoking history of 28 cpd for 38.5 years were given a standardised interview which assessed smoking history, baseline smoking levels, and SCT predictor variables (outcome expectancies, self-efficacy expectations, motivational factors). Smoking behavior was reassessed at 1- and 3-month post-test. Hierarchical multiple regression analysis controlled for age, sex, baseline smoking and smoking history, found that self-efficacy was the only significant SCT predictor for reduced smoking. The other SCT variables hypothesised contributed to smoking reductions via their interaction with self-efficacy but not independent of it. Finally, it was observed that presentation of a standard educational package did not contribute significantly to reduce smoking, indicating that self-efficacy plays a larger role in behavior change than education.

108.   Haug, K., Aaro, L. E., & Fugelli, P. (1992). Smoking habits in early pregnancy and attitudes towards smoking cessation among pregnant women and their partners. Family Practice, 9(4), 494-499.

The study aimed to investigate smoking habits and attitudes amoung pregnant smokers. The effect of partners' smoking habits on pregnant smokers were also assessed. In Norway, 398 general practitioners recorded the smoking habits of 2379 women at their first pregnancy check up. The sample contained 674 women aged between 18 and 34, who lived with a partner. Subjects smoked at least 5 cpd for the last 3 months before pregnancy and smoked at least 1 cpd at the first check up. These women were invited to participate in the smoking cessation study. Some subjects refused to participate leaving 530 subjects in the sample. The subjects completed a questionnaire about smoking habits and attitudes towards their own and their partner's smoking during pregnancy.

Results showed that of the 337 who had had a previous pregnancy, 14% smoked during at least 1 former pregnancy, 6% had reduced their cigarette consumption and 26% had remained unaltered. During the study, 93% recognised smoking as a problem, 97% indicated intentions to change smoking habits, 62% indicated intentions to quit and 11% did not expect to be able to change. Negative attitude to smoking during pregnancy was significantly higher among subjects who were encouraged to stop smoking and subjects who expected partner support. A mean reduction in cigarette consumption from before pregnancy to the first medical check up was 31%. The mean cigarette consumption was higher in women in their first pregnancy. They also showed greater reductions by the first follow-up and had greater partner support than women with previous pregnancies. It was concluded that pregnancy is an ideal time to illicit changes in smoking behavior, and strategies to achieve reduction or cessation should be aimed at both partners.

109.   Shiffman, S., Zettler-Segal, M., Kassel, J., Paty, J., Benowitz, N. L., &
        O'Brien, G. (1992). Nicotine elimination and tolerance in non-
        dependent cigarette smokers. Psychopharmacology, 109 (4), 449-456.

        Ten regular smokers (RS) smoked an average of 20-40 cpd and 10
        chippers (CH) averaged no more than 5 cpd and smoked at least 4
        days per week were each paid $100 for their participation. Groups
        were matched on gender, age, number of years smoking and nicotine
        delivery of cigarettes. It was hypothesised that slow nicotine elimina-
        tion and/or reduced nicotine tolerance underlies CH ability to maintain
        low levels of smoking. Elimination kinetics and pharmacodynamics of
        nicotine were studied in CH and matched RS by observing plasma
        nicotine levels and cardiovascular responses for several hours after
        uniform doses of tobacco smoke were delivered. Results found that
        CH eliminated nicotine at the same rate as RS. The result showed that
        CH do not smoke to maintain minimum levels of nicotine. Therefore it
        was suggested that CH are not motivated to smoke by withdrawal
        avoidance. The authors commented on the small and highly selected
        sample and the problems caused by generalisation. Physiological data
        was discussed in detail and suggestions as to why CH maintain a low
        smoking rate were explored.

110.   Haug, K., Aaro, L. E., & Fugelli, P. (1993). Smoking habits in early
        pregnancy related to age of smoking debut. Family Practice, 10(1), 66-
        69.

        The study investigated the relationship between age of smoking onset
        and cigarette consumption in early pregnancy. A sample of 530
        women were aged between 18 and 34 years, who lived with a partner,
        and were in the first trimester of pregnancy, were asked to complete a
        questionniare. Subjects smoked at least five cpd for three months
        before pregnancy and at least one cpd at the first medical check up in
        pregnancy. The questionnaire focussed on age of smoking onset,
        smoking habits before and during the current and any previous preg-
        nancies and smoking habits of significant others. Age of onset of daily
        smoking was before 15 years (group A) for 21%, between 15 and 16
        years (group B) for 45%, and 17 years or older (group C) for 34%.
        Mean smoking rate before pregnancy was 12.8 cpd. Women in group
        A smoked more cpd before pregnancy in both mean consumption and
        fraction of heavy smokers, and were still smoking more at their first
        medical check up in pregnancy than groups B and C. A quarter of the
        women in group A and B had reduced consumption by more than 10
        cpd compared with 11% in group C. Women in group A reported less
        reduction during previous pregnancies than groups B and C. In group

A, 59% reported the smoking habits of their best friend was an important influence of their own onset compared with 41% in group C. All three groups reported a reduction of 30% after getting pregnant, which indicated that even the "most addicted" women are capable of reducing cigarette consumption during pregnancy. It was predicted that smoking onset at an early age resulted in less success in maintained reductions throughout the pregnancy. Strategies to reduce smoking during pregnancy were presented.

111. Kinne, S., Kristal, A. R., White, E., & Hunt, J. (1993). Work-site smoking policies: Their population impact in Washington State. American Journal of Public Health, 83 (7), 1031-1033.

A population based random digit dialling telephone survey in 1989-1990 contacted 1228 employed adults in Washington State. Smoking habits and history followed by occupation, tenure, workplace smoking restrictions and the effect of smoking restrictions on their smoking behavior both on and off the job were recorded. Eighty-one percent of men and 91% of women reported work-site smoking restrictions. Respondents employed in no smoking work-sites were less likely to be current smokers and more likely to be never smokers than workers in less restricted settings. Male smokers in settings with smoking policies smoked fewer cigarettes on workdays than non-workdays compared to their unrestricted counterparts. Results suggested that 43% of employed male smokers and 74% of employed female smokers reduced their smoking on workdays and 48% of men and 53% of women attributed reduction in overall smoking to worksite policies. It was concluded that worksite smoking policies although intended to protect against smoke exposure, may also reduce employee smoking.

112. Hajek, P., West, R. & Wilson, J. (1995). Regular smokers, lifetime very light smokers, and reduced smokers: Comparison of psychosocial and smoking characteristics in women. Health Psychology, 14 (3), 195-201.

Stable very light smokers were compared to stable regular smokers from a population of mothers of newborn infants and followed-up for one year. Very light smokers (VLS) were defined as smoking more than 1 cigarette per week but less than 5 cpd without increasing smoking behavior of 5 cpd for more than 6 weeks per year. The VLS were divided according to smoking history, into lifetime very light smokers (VLS/L), as described above, and reduced smokers (VLS/R), those who had at one time smoked more than 10 cpd for more than 4 months. Regular smokers (RS) were defined as those who smoked at least 15 cpd without reduction for more than 6 weeks in the previous year. Sixty-one VLS and 61 RS made up the sample. Subjects were visited at their home for a 1-hour interview which involved a saliva sample (for cotinine analysis), collection of a 7 day smoking diary and questionaries including   General Smoking Questionnaire (GSQ), Smoking Motivation Questionnaire (SMQ), Smoking Career Questionnaire, Family Smoking History Questionnaire, Eysenck Personality Inventory and Subjective Effects of Smoking Questionnaire. Subjects weight, heart rate, breath holding endurance and end-expired CO measures were taken before a cigarette, and then after a cigarette. Results showed that VLS were not novice smokers or felt pressure to limit their smoking. VLS/R were very similar to VLS/L in many respects with VLS and RS differing in several important aspects including educational level and familial smoking patterns. VLS were found to use smoking as a mainly social activity with a large emphasis on pleasurable relaxation.

113.   Owen, N., Kent, P., Wakefield, M., & Roberts, L. (1995). Low-rate smokers. Preventive Medicine, 24, 80-84.

Chippers are described as smokers who maintain low levels of daily cigarette consumption and who do not appear to be addicted to nicotine. The prevalence and characteristics associated with chippers was examined from a population-representative survey. Data was collected by personal interview conducted in the homes of 3379 people over 15 years of age. A range of sociodemographic, contextual, cognitive and smoking behavior variables were examined. Of the people surveyed, 839 were current smokers and 697 of these were over 20 years of age and had been smoking for more than 2 years. Of this sample, 8.2% smoked 5 or less cpd and had a mean age of 38.7 years. Over 75% had smoked regularly for more than 10 years, averaging 3.45 cpd. The chippers were more likely to perceive quitting as not very difficult, smoked their first cigarette more than 30 minutes after waking, bought smaller packets of cigarettes and were not given cessation advise by a doctor. No evidence was found to support the theory that chippers were more likely than regular smokers to work in places with smoking bans.

114.   Severson, H. H., Andrews, J. A., Lichtenstein, E., Wall, M., & Zoref, L. (1995). Predictors of smoking during and after pregnancy: A survey of mothers of newborns. Preventive Medicine, 24, 23-28.

The study examines data from a large cohort of women two weeks postpartum and provides an overview of smoking and abstinent behavior during pregnancy and immediately after birth. Smoking history, psychosocial characteristics and demographic predictors were collected of smokers who quit, relapsed, reduced use or smoked at their usual rate during pregnancy. Data was collected from 13 495 mothers at the healthy newborns first pediatrician visit, usually at 2 weeks old. The subjects had a mean age of 28.21 years with 89.5% high school graduates, 30.4% college graduates, and 86.5% Caucasian Results found the sample when compared to the larger population were older and better educated but with similar racial/ethnic background.

Twenty-one point five percent reported smoking prior to pregnancy and the smokers tended to be younger, less well educated, and more likely to have consumed alcohol in the week prior to enrolment than non-smokers. Of the smokers, 35.4% reported continued abstinence, 6.4% quit for pregnancy but relapsed, 52% had reduced intake during pregnancy and 6.3% had remained unchanged. The continued abstainers appeared to be younger, better educated, smoked less prior to pregnancy, less often had a partner or others in the household smoke, and rarely or never allowed smoking in the house themselves. The opposite was true for those whose smoking behavior remained unchanged during pregnancy. Age and the amount smoked prior to pregnancy were related to smoking reductions during pregnancy. Women who reduced smoking during pregnancy were also less ready to quit than women who quit during pregnancy but relapsed.

115.   Secker-Walker, R. H., Soloman, L. J., Flynn, B. S., Skelly, J. M., & Mead, P. B. (1998). Reducing smoking during pregnancy and post partum: Physician's advice supported by individual counselling. Preventive Medicine, 27, 422-430.

The study assessed the effectiveness of structured physician's advice and referral to individual counselling with pregnant women. Women smoking one or more cpd at their first physician visit were randomly assigned to usual care (C) or physician advcice and referral to counselling (I) groups. All women completed baseline questionnaires, breath CO level was measured, and received a brief standardized health risk message about smoking during pregnancy from a nurse. The I group contained 135 women with mean age of 22.6 years, and the C group contained 141 women wth mean age 22.5 years. The mean cpd prior to pregnancy was 26.1 and 25.1 cpd, and the cpd at first visit was 13.4 and 11.8 cpd for the I and C groups respectively. The C group received information regarding the dangers of smoking during pregnancy from their physician, and arranged either a date to quit completely, a date to quit for 24 hours, or a date to halve their cigarette consumption. The I group women were immediately referred to a smoking cessation counsellor for individual counselling. This procedure was repeated at the 2nd, 3rd, and 5th visits, and at the 36th week visit. Self-reported smoking status information and expired air CO levels were measured for the C group at the 2nd visit and 36th week visit. Self-reported smoking status information and expired air CO levels were measured in the I group at every visit. Urinary cotinine analysis was conducted at the 1st and 36th week visit, and all women were followed-up one year postpartum. No significant differences were found in cessation at the 36th week or 1-year follow-up. The I group significantly reduced/stopped smoking at their 2nd visit, 36th week visit, and 1-year follow-up compared to the control group. It is concluded that physician advice and individual counselling shows promise in reducing smoking during preganacy and post partum.

5

SMOKER x TREATMENT

116.   Suedfeld, P. & Ikard, F. F. (1974). Use of sensory deprivation in facilitation the reduction of cigarette smoking. Journal of Consulting and Clinical Psychology, 42(6), 888-895.

The study examined the effectiveness of sensory deprivation in the reduction and/or cessation among subjects who were heavily psychologically committed to smoking. Thirty-five addicted and 42 pre-addictive smokers (categorized by results from Tomkins-Ikard Smoking Scale) had an average smoking history of 32 cpd for 15 years. They were equally split with males and females from a range of occupations, educational levels and backgrounds. Subjects were randomly assigned to one of four conditions: Sensory Deprivation - messages (SD-M) which consisted of 24 hours of sensory deprivation with one message presented every 1½ hours; Sensory deprivation - no messages (SD) consisting of 24 hours of SD; Messages - no sensory deprivation (M) where subjects remained confined at home, close to a phone through which messages were given, 1 every 1.5 hours for 24 hours; and NO messages - no sensory deprivation (C) where subjects were told to seek other forms of treatment. The sensory deprivation was administered in a shielded, dark, sound-reducing chamber with only a hospital bed and chemical toilet, with water and vanilla flavoured diet food available via tubes when lying on the bed. Subjects were dressed in simple garments and told to lie still for 24 hours.

The mean cigarette consumption was reduced to approximately one half, and over a quarter of subjects remained abstinent 1 year after a single session. SD and SD-M maintained a reduction of 50% of baseline at 12-month follow-up while the M group relapsed to 90% of baseline. Type of smoker (addicted vs pre-addicted) gave no significant interactions with other variables. Subjects who maintained a reduction of 1 to 2 thirds of baseline reported a decrease or elimination of symptoms like chronic coughing and an increased sense of well being. Time and cost advantages of SD and explanations for success were discussed.

117.   Gaston, C. D., & Hutzell, R. R. (1976). Hypnosis to reduce smoking in a deaf patient. American Journal of Clinical Hypnosis, 19(2), 125-127.

The study reported the procedure of hypnosis used to reduce smoking in a deaf person. Previously- reported procedures of pantomime, sign language and stroking techniques were discussed. Induction through lip reading was presented as a technique, which closely parallels the common verbal induction techniques. The patient was a 51 years old deaf male suffering from emphysema and bronchitis and smoking a baseline of over three packs of cigarettes a day. The patient was told to fix his gaze upon the therapist's lips. After an hypnotic state was achieved the therapist suggested the patient would substitute his desire for cigarettes to a desire for other orally stimulating materials. He was told not to smoke for certain portions of each hour of the day. Results show that daily cigarette consumption decreased from 60 to almost none and the patient averaged less than 2 cpd for 9 months follow-up. Difficulties and variations of the hypnotic procedure were discussed.

118.   Edinger, J. D., Nelson, W. M., Davidson, K. M., & Wallace, J. (1978). Modification of smoking behaviors in a correctional institution. Journal of Clinical Psychology, 34 (4), 991-998.

Two studies in a prison setting were used to determine the effectiveness of self-control procedures to reduce cigarette smoking with institutionalized subjects. In Study 1, 14 male inmates with an average age of 23.5 years reported smoking for an average of 9.4 years. They volunteered to try to quit or reduce their smoking. The program was administered to 9 subjects who averaged 18.24 cpd. Treatment consisted of four, 90-minute weekly group sessions and presented techniques of self-monitoring, changing criterion goal setting (for gradual reduction), aversive imagery, positive self-statements, muscle relaxation training, substitution, mini-goals, stimulation narrowing and self-reward/punishment. Only six subjects completed treatment. Pearson product moment correlations found a strong relationship between actual smoking rates and goals set by the subjects. It was suggested that the changing criterion design assisted in smoking reductions. The average post-treatment and follow-up levels of smoking were 45.6% and 38.1% of baseline respectively. These reductions from baseline were reported significant using an analysis of variance. The large dropout rate, problems of generalization, differences in goals and differences in self-control techniques used by the subjects who completed Study 1 were the focus of Study 2.

Twenty-four inmates, 23 cigarette smokers and one pipe smoker, commenced treatment and averaged 15.58 cpd/8.58 bowls of pipe tobacco per day. Subjects were dichotomized into internals and externals from scores on the Rotter I-E scale and were randomly assigned to either therapist or client goal-setting of gradual reductions. Written contracts were used to discourage dropouts. Nineteen subjects completed treatment and achieved significant smoking reductions of 44.5% post-treatment and 37.0% at follow-up. Analysis revealed the more helpful components of the program, a lower dropout rate than Study 1 and self-control treatment success with a pipe smoker.

119.   Ashton, H., Stepney, R., & Thompson, J. W. (1979). Self-titration by cigarette smokers. British Medical Journal, 2, 357-360.

The self-titration of nicotine content was analyzed in smokers of different strength cigarettes as an important contributor in planning and evaluating the effects of safer smoking strategies. Twelve middle tar/nicotine smokers had a mean age of 28.6 years and mean smoking history of 22.5 cpd for at least 2 years. Cigarettes and expenses for attendance were provided. Cigarettes were presented in unbranded packs. Subjects smoked their usual brand for three weeks. Group 1 then smoked cigarettes of high nicotine (1.84 mg) for six weeks followed by low nicotine (0.6 mg) for two weeks while group 2 smoked cigarettes of low nicotine for six weeks followed by high nicotine for two weeks. Weekly cigarette consumption, puffing behavior, butt analysis, plasma and urine nicotine concentration, blood carboxy-haemoglobin (COHb), heart rate, fingertip temperature, subjective rating scores and personality characteristics were measured. Butt analysis showed mouth nicotine intake was greater with high nicotine cigarettes and lower with low nicotine cigarettes than usual brand. The difference between high and low nicotine brands was highly significant. Plasma nicotine and blood COHb concentrations showed that medium nicotine smokers adjusted smoking topography to obtain a greater than expected nicotine yield from weaker cigarettes and a less than expected yield from stronger cigarettes indicating self-titration on nicotine and CO. Data showed compensation in nicotine and CO of about 66% of standard when switching to either high or low nicotine cigarettes.

120.   Barmann, B. C., Burnett, G. F., Malde, S. R., & Zinik, G. (1980). Token reinforcement procedures for reduction of cigarette smoking in a psychiatric outpatient clinic. Psychological Reports, 47, 1245-1246.

The study used an ABAB design to assess the effects of token reinforcement on the reduction of cigarette smoking on psychiatric outpatient clinics. Thirty outpatients averaged a hospitalization period of 7.5 years before becoming an outpatient. They had a mean age of 45 years and all except one were current smokers. Cigarette smoking was determined by the number of butts found after the departure of the subjects each day. All subjects remained inside the center until the usual departure time, all ward attendants were non-smokers and visitors were not permitted to smoke. During the treatment weeks subjects who were not smoking were randomly awarded lapel buttons saying "Thank you for not smoking". Different staff members awarded tokens randomly, at unannounced times of the day. On specified days the tokens were exchanged for merchandize. Baseline smoking was assessed in week 1 followed by 1 week of treatment. The treatment was withdrawn in week 3 and returned in week 4. Follow-up assessment occurred at 3-, 6-, 9-, and 12-months post-treatment. Baseline measures counted an average of 255 butts per day averaging 14.2 cpd per outpatient. A sharp reduction occurred in week 2, to an average of 4.97 cpd per outpatient. The reduction relapsed to near baseline during week 3. In week 4 there were reductions to near 4 cpd per outpatient. Twenty-one outpatients reduced smoking by over 70% with 3 stopping completely. Follow-up showed reductions were maintained. This method of reducing smoking behavior was described as easily administered, cost-effective and successful.

121.   Hymowitz, N. (1982). The Multiple Risk Factor Intervention Trial: A four-year evaluation. International Journal of Mental Health, 11(3), 44-67.

Elevated serum cholesterol, cigarette smoking, and hypertension were identified as the most important and modifiable risk factors for coronary heart disease. This study reported the progress after 4 years of an ongoing 6-year Multiple Risk Factor Intervention Trial (MR FIT). The primary objective was to discover if a group of men at high risk of death by Coronary Heart Disease (CHD) gave a reduced mortality after intervention to reduce the three outlined risk factors. Twelve thousand, eight hundred and sixty-six men aged 35-57 who were in the upper 10-15% of coronary risk due to the presence of risk factors volunteered for the study. They did not have diagnosed CHD. Subjects were randomly assigned into two groups. A special intervention group (SI) involved risk factor modification was supplied to produce a 10% reduction in baseline serum cholesterol, and a 10% reduction in baseline diastolic blood pressure. A 25% reduction in cpd was introduced to heavy smokers, a 40% reduction in cpd was introduced to moderate smokers, and a 55% reduction in cpd was introduced for light smokers. The usual care group (UC) was referred to their usual source of medical care. Data were collected annually for UC, and every 4 months for SI groups. Smoking cessation at the time of the 4-year follow-up was approximately 40% of SI and 20% of UC groups. No smoking reduction data were reported. The blood pressure (systolic and diastolic) at 4 years had reduced in both SI and UC to lower than anticipated levels. A reduction in serum cholesterol levels for UC subjects was reported. It did not reach the goals set. Mortality and morbidity data were expected at 6-year follow-up.

122.   O'Conner, K. P. & Stravynski, A. (1982) Evaluation of a smoking typology by use of a specific behavioral substitution method of self-control. Behavior Research and Therapy, 20 (3), 279-288.

The aim of the study was to test the efficacy of situational smoking typology in designing reduction strategies. Twenty-four subjects were allocated into high and low activity groups based on the results from a Situational Smoking Questionnaire. The high activity group was subdivided into those people who smoked under emotional stress or to aid concentration. The low activity group was subdivided into people who smoked to relieve boredom or who smoked to relax. Subjects were then randomly allocated to one of three treatment groups. Relaxation, coping, and distraction activities were presented in the Behavioral Substitution group (BS), and rehearsed according to which activity group the subject originated. The generalized coverant group (GC) discussed generalized beliefs about smoking rather than situational beliefs with no specific behavior instruction. The third group was a control group who self-monitored smoking behavior over the treatment period. All subjects self-monitored smoking for 7 days, completed for treatment sessions and a 2 and 8-month follow-up. Both treatment groups showed a reduction in smoking post-treatment with the BS group significantly lower post-treatment and at follow-up (approximately 19 cpd at baseline to 7 cpd post-treatment to 5 cpd at 8 month follow up). Attitude measures changed most significantly in the GC group. This treatment appeared to increase motivation to reduce smoking. The inclusion of a differential situational model of smoking effects in cessation programs was discussed.

123.   Stitzer, M. L., & Bigelow, G. E. (1982). Contingent reinforcement for reduced carbon monoxide levels in cigarette smokers. Addictive Behaviors, 7(4), 403-412.

The effect of contingent reinforcement (monetary rewards) for reduced carbon monoxide (CO) levels in regular smokers who were not planning on reducing or quitting smoking was assessed. Eleven subjects averaged 38 years had a mean smoking history of 22 cpd for 20.5 smoking years. Subjects were given free cigarettes throughout the study. They self-monitored smoking for 3 weeks and were visited at work for 3 weeks to obtain an expired air sample for CO analysis. At each visit, self-monitoring cards, empty cigarette packs and unused cigarettes were collected. A supply of cigarettes for use until the next visit was distributed. During week 2, $5 was awarded to subjects whose CO level was 50% below the average reading obtained from week 1. Results showed that CO levels reduced during the contingent reinforcement intervention often failed to return to baseline levels when the reinforcement was withdrawn. Daytime cigarette consumption averaged 11.3 during baseline, reduced to 8.2 during contingent reinforcement and increased to 9.9 post-treatment. The mean evening cigarette rate remained constant at 10 throughout the study. A similar pattern of CO levels and daytime cigarette frequency was observed for mean time since last cigarette prior to the afternoon visit for CO measure. It was concluded that contingent reinforcement was an effective method to reduce cigarette smoking. Expired air CO level has an appropriate tool for analysis of recent cigarette smoking.

124.   Strecher, V. J., Becker, M. H., Kirscht, J. P., Eraker, S. A., & Graham-Tomasi, R. P. (1985). Psychosocial aspects of changes in cigarette-smoking behavior. Patient Education and Counseling, 7, 249-262.

This study examined the relationship between patients' perception of susceptibility to illness, self-efficacy, anxiety, and social support, with changes in smoking behavior. Patients of a Veterans Administration Medical Center (VAMC) were given either practitioner initiated minimal contact smoking intervention or a usual care. Of the 213 inpatients and outpatients approached for treatment, 30% reported not wishing to stop smoking or refused treatment. Seventy-two male patients accepted the smoking cessation intervention with 74 in the usual care control group. Patients were assigned (by time period) to an intervention or control group and completed a questionnaire that assessed the number of cigarettes smoked and characteristics associated with smoking behavior or cessation. Smoking rate was also assessed at 3-months following discharge from the VAMC. Intervention consisted of three components: consultation from a health practitioner, a self-help smoking cessation kit, and incentives to comply with the self-help kit. The first series of activities in the kit was completed. The patient and the remainder of the diary were to be completed on their own, reinforced by weekly telephone calls from the practitioner. A free State lottery ticket was given for each week of the diary completed.

Of the 146 subjects, 119 were successfully recontacted 3-months following hospital discharge. Results showed efficacy expectations for quitting smoking, and perceived susceptibility to illness due to smoking, was significantly predictive of changes in smoking at follow-up. Subjects with high-perceived susceptibility and high expectations of efficacy were far more likely to have reduced smoking at 3-months than any other group. Subjects who reported high susceptibility and low efficacy were least likely to reduce smoking. Also, subjects in this group were most likely to be found in the least effective response condition - "learned helplessness". No direct relationships were found between anxiety or social support and changes in amount smoked. It was noted however that people with high reported levels of anxiety had on average low levels of self-efficacy. It was concluded that the practitioner could adopt optimal consultation styles based on the psychological state of the patient. This would help to develop a tailored intervention strategy.

125.   Kabela, E., & Andrasik, F. (1988). Behavioral and biochemical effects of gradual reductions in cigarette yields in pregnant and nonpregnant smokers. Addictive Behaviors, 13 (3), 231-243.

Pregnant smokers have received scant attention in the smoking cessation and risk reduction literature. It was suggested that pregnancy might be an optimal time for cessation or reduction intervention due to the dual responsibility for the health of both mother and foetus. Twelve female smokers, six pregnant (P) and six non-pregnant (GNP) smokers were included in a study with a focus of reduction not cessation. Subjects were asked to smoke at their usual rate during four sessions. Subjects smoked their usual brand in session 1 then switched to a brand approximately 0.3 mg lower in nicotine per cigarette for two weeks before the next session. Reductions continued so that by session 4 subjects were smoking between 0.6 and 1.2 mg of nicotine per cigarette lower than their usual brand. Cigarette and puff frequency, cigarette duration/length, and carbon monoxide (CO) thiocyanate (SCN) levels were recorded during the sessions. Both P and NP smokers showed no significant change in puff or cigarette frequencies during brand switching. Both groups showed significantly shorter cigarette duration with the low yield brands. No between-group differences were observed. Both groups showed a significant decreasing trend in daily nicotine rate, but no significant change in daily smoking rate. P smokers showed a tendency to have lower and less variable COHb and SCN levels than NP smokers. Both group means of COHb levels did not drop below the minimal risk level. It was concluded that P smokers not interested in quitting may be more suited to a controlled smoking program (which reduced nicotine and tar intake by brand switching).

126. Hartman, N., Jarvik, M. E., & Wilkins, J. N. (1989). Reduction of cigarette smoking by use of a nicotine patch. Archives of General Psychiatry, 46(3), 289.

The use of transdermal nicotine patches to reduce smoking in hospitalized psychiatric patients was presented. Three moderate smokers of one to two packs per day for at least 10 years participated in a single-blind study. Either 24µl of a solution containing 30% nicotine base or water (the control) was placed and covered on the non-dominant forearm in two separate 7-hour sessions at a 1-week interval. Patients were then allowed unlimited access to a standard popular brand of cigarette. They were instructed to forget the patch and smoke normally. All butts were saved (for cigarette count) and a 7-hour urine sample was collected. Cigarette consumption was substantially decreased in each patient during the treatment time when the nicotine patch was worn, and urine output also decreased. It was concluded that transdermally-administered nicotine might be used to reduce the number of cigarettes smoked. The authors suggested that the success of this pilot study encouraged further full-scale studies.

127. Shiffman, S., Fischer, L. B., Zettler-Segal, M., & Benowitz, N. L. (1990). Nicotine exposure among nondependent smokers. Archives of General Psychiatry, 47(4), 333-336.

Nicotine and cotinine analysis of stable non-dependent very light smokers (Chippers) and dependent smokers were assessed. Compensation with nicotine absorption of chippers was investigated. Ten chippers who smoked no more than 5 cpd for at least 4 days each week, gave a mean age of 38.3 years, had a mean of 17.8 smoking years and smoked an average of 3.9 cpd of 0.79 mg nicotine. Twelve dependent smokers who smoked between 20 and 40 cpd and met the criteria for tobacco dependence also served as subjects. They had a mean age of 34.8 years, mean smoking history of 23.8 cpd of 0.82-mg nicotine for 19.2 smoking years. Venous blood samples were taken immediately before and after a cigarette of usual brand smoked at their own pace. Breath carbon monoxide (CO) levels were measured with the number of puffs taken, and the smoking rate on the test and preceding day. Analysis showed chippers inhaled tobacco smoke and absorbed as much nicotine as dependent smokers, both in the laboratory and in the field. Chippers nicotine exposure was then compared to regular smokers (whose smoking was temporarily restricted to 5 cpd).

Ten subjects smoked an average of 38.4 cpd of 1.1-mg nicotine for 22.5 smoking years and had a mean age of 39.4 years. The subjects smoked normally in the first session then smoked 15, 10 and 5 cpd in the subsequent sessions. Venous blood samples were taken at different times. Results indicated that the dependent smokers were compensating by extracting more nicotine from each cigarette, and that chippers had significantly lower blood cotinine concentrations than heavy smokers when restricted to 5 cpd. It was concluded that chippers did not compensate for their low smoking rate by extracting more nicotine per cigarette.

128.   Pomerleau, O. F., Pomerleau, C. S., Morrell, E. M., & Lowenbergh, J. M. (1991). Effects of fluoxetine on weight gain and food intake in smokers who reduce nicotine intake. Psychoneuroendocrinology, 16 (5), 433-440.

Weight gain was observed not only in people who abstained completely but also in smokers who substantially reduced cigarette consumption. Fluoxetine is a selective serotonin uptake inhibitor. It has been reported to decrease eating and produce weight loss. The effects have been linked to a reduction in 'carbohydrate craving'. This study was a placebo-controlled clinical trial of fluoxetine after behavioral smoking cessation treatment to examine how fluoxetine affected weight and intake of food when nicotine intake was decreased. Eleven subjects in the placebo group and 10 in the fluoxetine group averaged 47.4 and 43.9 years and 27.5 and 30.0 cpd respectively. The subjects participated in a minimal behavioral intervention for smoking. It was designed for quit smoking subject. All subjects reduced cotinine levels to less than 50% of baseline, and attended a pre- and post- nicotine reduction lunch session of cheese pizza and chocolate bars, 70 days apart. Placebo subjects gained significantly more weight (+3.3 kg) than fluoxetine (-0.6 kg). Changes in eating showed a significant positive correlation with changes in weight in individuals. Fluoxetine may have prevented weight gain by decreasing food consumption. The data did not show whether fluoxetine differentially affected intake of sweet-tasting food. It was concluded that for smokers, whose fear of weight gain was a motive of continued smoking, fluoxetine could be used as a preventative treatment to achieve smoking cessation or reduction without weight gain.

129.   Withey, C. H., Papacosta, A. O., Swan, A. V., Fitzsimons, B. A., Ellard, G. A., Burney, P. G. J., Colley, J. R. T., & Holland, W. W. (1992). Respiratory effects of lowering tar and nicotine levels of cigarettes smoked by young male middle tar smokers. II. Results of a randomised controlled trial. Journal of Epidemiology and Community Health, 46, 281-285.

The study investigated the effect of lowered tar and nicotine levels of cigarettes on respiratory health of the smoker. Middle tar smokers were randomly assigned to smoke middle tar/middle nicotine (1), low tar/middle nicotine (2), or low tar/low nicotine (3) cigarettes for six-months. Respiratory health was analyzed by respiratory symptoms, peak expiratory flow rates and nicotine inhalation. Results showed little differences between the three groups for the duration of the study. Urinary nicotine analysis indicated subjects in each group adjusted their smoking to maintain nicotine levels similar to baseline. Group 3 and 2 had calculated tar reductions of 14 and 18% respectively. It was concluded that due to smoking compensation, only modest reductions in tar intake could be achieved by reducing the tar and nicotine yield of cigarettes smoked. Reductions of 18% in tar intake failed to show any effect on respiratory health measures.

130.   Haug, K., Fugelli, P., Aaro, L. E., & Foss, O. P. (1994). Is smoking intervention in general practice more successful among pregnant than non-pregnant women? Family Practice, 11(2), 111-116.

The study was aimed to evaluate the extent to which a simple inter-vention program affected long- term smoking behavior in pregnant (P) and non-pregnant (NP) women. The intervention was implemented by general practitioners (GP) during medical consultations. Of the 2379 P women available, 674 had smoked at least 5 cpd for the last 3 months before pregnancy and at least 1 cpd at the first check up. Of these P women, 252 were subjects in the intervention group (I) and 98 in the control group (C), and 163 NP women served as subjects in the I group and 111 in the C group. At the first consultation, women in the I group were given verbal information about the health hazards of smoking. They were advised how to stop and how to avoid relapse. Special information was given to P women about "the smoking foetus". At the end of the first consultation a 5-page flipover and an 8-page booklet (a separate one for P and NP women) was distributed to all I subjects. They were invited to consult with their GP after 1-, 6-, 12- and 18-months to discuss progress and problems. C subjects received no advice on smoking, or flipovers or books. At the first consultation all subjects completed a questionnaire and blood test. At 12 months they had another blood test, and at 18 months a follow-up postal questionnaire.

Results showed 10% of P women and 12% of NP women in the I group were abstinent, compared to 5% of P women and 6% of NP women in the C group. Relapse occurred so that by the 18 month follow-up only 6% of P and 5 % of NP I women and 1% of NP C women remained abstinent. Cigarette reductions were reported by 25% of P and 34% of NP women. Intervention helped cessation of both P and NP women and reductions of NP women. It was concluded that more effective low cost intervention programs designed for P women should be studied.

131.   Valbo, A., & Eide, T. (1996). Smoking cessation in pregnancy: The effect of hypnosis in a randomized study. Addictive Behaviors, 21(1), 29-35.

The effect of hypnosis as a smoking reduction/cessation intervention method was assessed on women still smoking at the 18th week of pregnancy. The intervention group (H) contained 52 women with mean age 27.9 years, and the control group (C) contained 78 women with mean age 26.5 years. No significant differences between groups were found on age, education, cpd prior to pregnancy or at time of delivery, interest or presumed difficulty in quitting, or number of previous quit attempts. The C group received usual care, while the H group received 2 sessions of hypnosis over 4 weeks. Each session of 45 minutes included a conventional trance induction. A tape was played emphasizing the unpleasant effects of smoking and reaffirming quit intentions, and relaxation techniques were practised. Self-hypnosis to combat cravings was taught. Results showed the intervention had no significant effects on smoking cessation or reduction. A 10% cessation rate in both groups was found, and 42% of the H group, 31% of the C group reduced smoking. It was concluded that the present clinical and statistical evidence did not support the use of hypnosis in smoking reduction/cessation.

6

REVIEWS

132.   Hunt, W. A., & Matarazzo, J. D. (1973). Three years later: Recent developments in the experimental modification of smoking behavior. Journal of Abnormal Psychology, 81, 107-114.

Hunt and Matarazzo suggested the general relapse rate over time of a group of subjects who had successfully completed a treatment program to stop smoking could be plotted as a negatively accelerated curve, similar to the extinction curve in the learning literature. Most new non-smokers rapidly resumed smoking with graduated increments to baseline, typically reported as abstinence with relapse to baseline. If all new non-smokers were to be represented on a graph, a line could be drawn to indicate a trend where a large number relapse to baseline while a small number remain non-smokers, shown by the curve approaching an asymptote well above zero. The discovery of a typical, relatively common curve of smoking behavior could provide a reference line to evaluate new treatment programs. The amount and nature of the data needed in research studies to provide a reliable comparison was discussed.

Four suggestions were made to improve smoking treatment programs. More effective stimulus conditions would provide more generalization outside the laboratory. Hot, dry air and satiation were aversive consequences of smoking and therefore should improve aversive conditioning if used as a stimuli rather than electric shock. A combination of multiple techniques could help more people reduce the deterioration to baseline smoking (although making analysis for the experimenter more complex). Maintenance of behavior change should play a major role, instead of the whole emphasis on achieving the desired behavior goal. Lastly a more comprehensive human engineering approach would make the individual the focus of planning rather than the treatment program. Several models are proposed to explain the curve as a detailed discussion was developed to suggest why some people did resume smoking and others did not resume smoking.

133.   Hunt, W. A., & Bespalec, D. A. (1974). An evaluation of current methods of modifying smoking behavior. Journal of Clinical Psychology, 30, 431-438.

The study provided an evaluative review of methods to modify smoking behavior. Studies with no follow-up data, non-specific treatment or no follow-up periods, and all studies with a sample of one were excluded. Results for relapse after successful treatment (often abstinence) plotted a negatively accelerated curve over time that asymptotes well above zero. A curve for the percent reduction from baseline smoking was very similar to the abstinence curve, that showed an initial decrease in smoking frequency, followed by relapse to an asymptote at around 40% of baseline. A summary of abstinence and reduction rates for aversive conditioning, drug therapy, education and group support, hypnosis, and reduction rates for behavior modification and miscellaneous were presented. The effects of investigator pre-selection of subjects and motivation of subjects on reported success and attrition rates were discussed.

134.   Russell, M. (1974) Realistic goals for smoking and health: A case for safer smoking. Lancet, 1, 254-258.

Russell proposed that a goal of safer smoking rather than a goal of no smoking was more realistic for most smokers. The realities of cigarette dependence were outlined to establish it as a life-long "dependence disorder". The crucial role of nicotine in cigarette dependence was also examined with an explanation of the modification of smoking products and behavior to regulate nicotine consumption. An historical example to illustrate this occurred with the spontaneous change to filter-tipped cigarettes without formal official effort. The reasons for the change were unclear. Filter-tipped cigarettes were reported as safer, and promoted the beginning of milder levels of nicotine, tar and carbon monoxide. The popularity of milder cigarettes demonstrated the consumers' goal of safer smoking rather than no smoking. This occurred at a time when cigarette education and quit programs were publicly advertised by agencies such as the Health Education Council. The failure of the anti-smoking approach was attributed to insufficient recognition of the nature of nicotine dependence. A more realistic goal was suggested with an aim towards achieving acceptably safe, light to moderate, controlled smoking.

135.   Thoresen, C. E., & Mahoney, M. J. (1974). Behavioral Self Control. USA: Holt Rinehart & Winston Inc.

The 144-page text defined, explained and explored the need for behavioral self-control and related techniques. A discussion of traditional and behavioral views, self-control criteria and general self-control strategies included environmental planning and behavioral programming. This was illustrated with case examples ranging from smoking and obesity to speech anxiety and test performance. Methodological techniques and problems in self-control research included controlling external factors and subject selection bias. Problems with expectation (both subject and experimenter) and self-observation occurred, as they were often ignored as variables that could produce a change in behavior. Experimental design in self-control research was listed, and success and failures of each was discussed. Chapters on self-observation, self-reward, self-punishment and covert self-control presented a discussion of successful and unsuccessful techniques and their underlying theories. The control (rather than the elimination) of smoking behavior was provided as an illustration of theories and procedures throughout the text.

136.   Bernstein, D. A., & McAlister, A. (1976). The modification of smoking behavior: Progress and problems. Addictive Behaviors, 1, 89-102.

Bernstein and McAlister presented an evaluative review of smoking modification research. The outcomes of controlled experimental research on smoking modification (mainly cessation) were reviewed, highlighting directions of future work. A range of approaches and techniques were categorized and success or failure in replication attempts was reported. Smoking cessation clinics varied in specific treatment techniques, and number and length of sessions. They tended to provide some combination of health information, encouragement, group therapy, moral support, social pressure and suggestions for resisting urges to smoke to a group of smokers who wanted help. Studies suggested that smoking reduction was temporary and with outcomes not much different from unaided efforts of self-help. Research was presented on a variety of anti-smoking drugs included lobeline sulphate. They were weak, temporary, with large placebo and other non-specific effects. Nicotine chewing gum has been associated with greater reductions in smoking, especially with heavy smokers. Nicotine was provided in a relatively safe form by eliminating tar, carbon monoxide, and other harmful consequences of inhalation. Hypnosis has been demonstrated to have little effect in smoking modification. Sensory deprivation could produce substantial reductions in smoking over periods as long as 2 years. Initially high abstinence rates however relapsed in the same pattern as many other interventions.

Social learning approaches focused on reductions of the probability of smoking behavior or increased probabilities of an alternate behavior to smoking. These included treatments such as systematic desensitization, punishment and aversive conditioning (electric shock, noise, warm smoky air, rapid smoking), stimulus control, and reinforcement of non-smoking. Multicomponent interventions included social learning interventions in combinations. These were designed to both suppress smoking behavior and to reinforce an adaptive alternative behavior. They often resulted in immediate abstinence/reduction rates with slower or less relapse than other interventions. Methodological considerations were discussed.

137.   Thornton, R. E. (Ed.). (1978). Smoking behaviour. Physiological and psychological influences. Edinburgh: Churchill Livingstone.

The book presented the 31 papers from the International Smoking Behaviour Conference held at Chelwood Vachery, Sussex, England in November 1977. The objectives of the conference were to explore the physiological and psychological effects of smoking which influenced smoking behavior and motivation in smokers and non-smokers. The intake of tar, nicotine and carbon monoxide from changes in cigarette design was also addressed. A wide range of smoking-related themes were presented. These included the effect of smoking on performance, the effect of smoking on the central nervous system, inter-smoker differences in smoking patterns, smokers' response on usual and altered cigarettes, the addictive nature of tobacco, and recommendations of objective measures.

138.   Wynder, E. L., & Hoffman, D. (1979). Tobacco and health: A societal challenge. New England Journal of Medicine, 300(16), 894-903.

A 3-directional approach was described as a necessary way to improve the societal problem of smoking and health. Youth anti-smoking programs were a preventative approach to combat early experimentation with tobacco and ultimately the acquisition of "smoking dependence". Two broad categories, an informational approach and a social and psychological approach, were used to group most youth anti-smoking programs. The first theorized that students provided with adequate information about hazards of smoking would choose to avoid it. The second category identified the nature of major social pressures to smoke and taught effective ways to cope with them. Anti-smoking programs for adults were diverse, with several options for smokers seeking assistance. Clinic approaches to smoking cessation included hypnosis, counseling, shock treatment, and rapid smoking. Other options included abrupt versus gradual quitting. The importance of maintenance was addressed. The third approach addressed smokers who could not (or would not) quit smoking. A discussion on the health benefits of a less harmful cigarette reports that while Chronic Obstructive Pulmonary Disease is non-reversible, its progression can be inhibited. In addition, risk of lung and larynx cancer, heart attacks, peripheral vascular disease, myocardial infarction, and chronic coughing can be reduced either gradually or in some cases almost immediately when smokers switch to less harmful cigarettes. Smoking and health was described as one of the largest challenges to the field of public health with a major impact on entire health care and economic systems.

139.   Gori, G. B., & Bock, F. G. (Eds.). (1980). A Safe Cigarette (Banbury Report 3). Cold Spring Harbor, U. S. A.:   Cold Spring Harbor Laboratory.

This 364-page text presented the proceedings of The Banbury Conference on Less Hazardous Cigarettes. This was attended by some of the leading scientists and experts in the field of cigarette smoking in 1979. The first section presented an introduction and epidemiological trends of cigarette smoking. General principles and future concerns of the Less Hazardous Cigarette were presented. Summaries of published data were presented on the long-term benefits of reduced tar and nicotine cigarettes, a comparison of number of cigarettes smoked to changes in tar and nicotine content, and the influence of tar exposure in lung cancer of males. An analysis of risk levels associated with cigarette smoking suggested a potential to reduce tobacco-related diseases as a public health problem.

The second section presented toxicological components of cigarette smoking with specific attention to the effects of nitrogen oxides, carbon monoxide, polonium 210, carcinogens, nicotine and N-nitros-amines. The effect of tobacco smoke on the lungs, cardiovascular diseases, and the Bronchial Epithelium was also outlined. The dialog of an open discussion on the achievements and future directions of a "less hazardous cigarette" by members of the conference was presented in the third section. The risk of lung cancer had been reduced for people who continued to smoke. This reduction was due to changes in cigarettes rather than smoking habits. Cigarettes in 1979 were "less hazardous" than cigarettes in 1959. Future changes to cigarettes without loss of acceptability and compensatory changes were also discussed. Construction and composition of cigarette smoke, reconstituted tobacco sheet, and agricultural, physical and structural modification to produce a less harmful cigarette were addressed in the fourth section. The last section presented the behavioral effects of switching to cigarettes with lower tar, nicotine and carbon monoxide and ethical concerns in the promotion of less hazardous cigarettes. The demographic and economic effects in the prevention of tobacco-related diseases were analyzed.

140.   Rickert, W. S. (1983). "Less hazardous" cigarettes: fact or fiction? New York State Journal of Medicine, 83(13), 1269-1272.

The "less hazardous" cigarette is based on a premise that reduced active ingredients in cigarettes could provide smokers who cannot or would not stop smoking with fewer smoking-related diseases. A review of the results of some investigations into the reduced health risk of the less hazardous cigarette was presented. Carbon monoxide (CO), tar, nicotine, aldehydes and hydrogen cyanide (HCN) were identified as some of the major components of tobacco smoke, which were biologically active and found in large amounts. During 1969-1978, significant reductions in tar, nicotine, HCN and aldehydes (but not CO yields) were reported in Canadian cigarettes. Tar and CO was further reduced by 1982. The authors suggested that change were a result of major changes in the construction of most cigarette brands. Consumer response to low tar brands has associated with increased sales in USA and Canada from 17% to 59% by 1982. Health consequences of smoking less hazardous cigarettes have received much research interest. It was reported that smokers of low tar/nicotine cigarettes have 20% lower lung cancer mortality than high tar cigarette smokers. No lowered risk of myocardial infarction or heart disease has been reported. The variable nature of human smoking behavior is unlike the consistent nature of smoking machines. Such machines measure the manufacturers' yields and have produced over or under compensation. This has resulted in conflict in yields of exposure to cigarette smoke components. The amount of hazard reduced by the less hazardous cigarette was highly variable and smoker-dependent.

141.   Miller, G. H. (1985). The "less hazardous" cigarette: a deadly delusion. New York State Journal of Medicine, 85(7), 313-317.

The establishment and development of the "less hazardous" cigarette was reviewed. The less hazardous cigarette was developed on the premise that most smokers cannot stop. The less hazardous cigarette should reduce the incidence of cigarette-related diseases. Early research was aimed at reductions in tar and nicotine to produce a less hazardous cigarette. Studies about the effects of the safer cigarettes generally showed lower mortality rates. The reliability of these studies has often been controversial, however. Some studies showed that low tar and nicotine cigarettes produced increased levels of carbon monoxide (CO) which could increase health risk. This conflicts with the premise of the less hazardous cigarette. The use of critical values have estimated safety levels of components of tobacco smoke like CO, tar, nitrogen oxides, nicotine, hydrogen cyanides and acrolein. Most levels have been based on speculation however rather than fact. Compensatory behaviors by smokers who changed to low tar/low nicotine cigarettes were also presented. The variability of human smoking compared to the apparent consistency of the smoking machine was highlighted. Effects of other components of tobacco smoke not publicized by the manufacturers or the media has challenged the efficiency of the less hazardous cigarette. The authors suggested that inaccurate information be used to advertise cigarettes. Research interest in the less hazardous cigarette should be redirected to education, skill development, and cessation programs.

142.   Grunberg, N. E., & Kozlowski, L. T. (1986). Alkaline therapy as an adjunct to smoking cessation programs. International Journal of Biosocial Research, 8(1), 43-52.

An overview of studies that assessed changes in cigarette smoking by manipulations of urinary pH was presented. Schachter (1977, cited in Grunberg & Kozlowski, 1986) proposed the amount of unmetabolized nicotine excreted from the body is related to urinary pH. Acidic urine was found to contain more unmetabolized nicotine than alkaline urine. Increases in the acidity of the urine would increase cigarette smoking (to replace lost nicotine) and decreases in the acidity of the urine would decrease cigarette smoking. Investigations have found similar biochemical results. The usefulness of alkaline therapy in smoking cessation was not confirmed (or even addressed). Many studies found it to have a modest effect to help smoking reductions. Analysis of the theory of urinary alkalinizers and cigarette smoking supported this conclusion. The theory suggested that urinary alkalization should decrease smoking as nicotine excretion was reduced. The plasma nicotine level was not depleted. Its usefulness for smoking cessation (when plasma and urinary nicotine is zero) was questionable. Both human and animal studies were reported.

143.   Alexander, L. L. (1987). Smoking cessation guidelines for the military health care provider. Military Medicine, 152(4), 175-178.

Cigarette smoking was identified as a detrimental health behavior, which caused premature mortality. The resulting involvement of health care resources produced large economic costs. The difficulty of smoking cessation required a significant behavioral change, personal commitment, and appropriate intervention techniques. Problems in the design and implementation of smoking cessation interventions were discussed.

Seven smoking cessation intervention areas were discussed. Self-help or self-management procedures were described as cost-effective intervention. Aversive procedures, such as electric shock, negative images, and cigarette smoke (rapid smoking and satiation) were aimed to reduce the reinforcing effect of smoking. It was paired with actual or imagined aversive stimuli. Gradual reduction strategies were aimed to reduce the smoker's physical dependence on nicotine to the point of complete cessation. Reductions occurred via nicotine fading, brand switching, or reduced smoking rate. Controlled smoking strategies were aimed to reduce the smoking to a less destructive rate, and to develop and maintain moderate smoking behavior. The long-term health effects of controlled smoking required further investigation.

Pharmacological strategies included drugs to alleviate smoking withdrawal, side effects (anticholinergices, sedatives, tranquilizers, sympathomimetics, and anticonvulsants). Agents were developed to help smokers abstain from smoking (nicotine substitutes like lobeline sulfate and nicotine gum, deterrents like astringent mouthwashes, and vegetable-based products). Altered states of consciousness like hypnosis and meditative states have also been included in smoking cessation programs. Comparisons of their effectiveness to other smoking cessation treatment were minimal. Multicomponent interventions have been designed to suppress smoking behavior and reinforce adaptive alternatives, combining aversive procedures, self-control, coverant control, social and material reinforcement, behavior modification, and many other cessation techniques. It was concluded that anti-smoking messages and proper referrals from health care workers could reduce health care costs and improve health.

144.   Donovan, D. M., & Marlatt, G. A. (Eds.). (1988). Assessment of Addictive Behaviors. New York: Guilford Press.

The book was aimed to provide an update and extension of previously reported information on the assessment of addictive behaviors. The book was comprised of 6 parts and was intended for use by students, clinicians and researchers. Part 1 provided an overview of the process of assessment for addictive behaviors. Parts 2,3 and 4 focused on drinking behavior, smoking behavior, and eating behavior respectively. Part 5 presented the assessment of other drugs of abuse, including cannabis, cocaine and heroin. A discussion of the relevance of the assessment process about aspects of treatment interventions for addictive behaviors was included in Part 6. Objective assessment procedures were required in smoking reduction or controlled smoking programs, as well as smoking cessation programs. Recommendations of biochemical indicators and physical procedures in monitoring progress and follow-up assessment were presented.

145.   Eriksen, M. P., & Kondo, A. T. (1989). Smoking cessation for cancer patients: Rationale and approaches. Special Issue: Cancer control. Health Education Research, 4 (4), 489-494.

The potential health benefits of: smoking cessation, smoking behavior reported before and after diagnosis and treatment, the factors associated with effective smoking cessation, and recommendations of reductions of smoking of cancer patients were reviewed and discussed. Tobacco users, who continued to smoke following initial treatment, especially for head and neck cancer patients, were at significantly higher risk of second primary tumors than smokers who quit or reduced tobacco consumption. Limited data were available on the smoking behavior of cancer patients before and after diagnosis/ treatment. Even minimal exposure of cancer patients to physician counseling produced high quit rates. Severity of the illness assisted in cessation success. Patients with more severe, late stage disease were most likely to have a greater motivation to quit. The therapeutic benefits were less for patients with early-stage disease. Many patients were not aware of the benefit of cessation following a cancer diagnosis. Cessation can provide the patient with feelings of hope and control over the disease, which can help recovery. Finally a series of recommendations for designing effective smoking cessation programs for cancer patients were discussed.

146.   Kozlowski, L. T. (1989). Reduction of tobacco health hazards in continuing users: Individual behavioral and public health approaches.

Special Issue: Nicotine uses ·and abuses: From brain probe to public health menace. Journal of Substance Abuse, 1(3), 345-357.

Less hazardous forms of tobacco use were presented for smokers who did not stop smoking. It was recognized that any tobacco product use was not "safe" or without risk. Nonetheless risk reduction had important implications for public health. Most studies did not find a "safe" level of smoking. It has been found however that disease rates increased as a function of increased smoking rates. It was suggested that small reductions by many individuals might be more important than large reductions by a few individuals, with regard to the impact on public health. Risk reductions were presented as a package rather than as single elements. Tobacco users should use the least amount of hazardous tobacco product. This could be achieved by reducing the number of cigarettes smoked each day, smoking lower yield cigarettes, keeping filter vents unblocked, changing to pipes or cigars which are less frequently inhaled, reducing the number of pipes or cigars each day, changing to smokeless tobacco products which do not contain the extra smoke toxins, limit the use of smokeless tobacco and finally change to nicotine containing gum. Many elements were involved in reducing risk factors. Alcohol consumption, other drug use, diet and exercise should be considered when tobacco use is reduced. Public health measures to promote less hazardous tobacco use should include decreased availability, increased penalties for sale to minors, regulate (or differentially tax) cigarettes according to pack size, differential taxation on tobacco products according to risk of disease, and social discouragement.

147.   Ney, T., & Gale, A. (Eds.). (1989). Smoking and Human Behavior. New York: Wiley.

The book was divided into four parts. Part 1 detailed the biochemical mechanisms of smoking. The effect of smoking on mood and behavior through the impact of nicotine on brain biochemistry was explored. The addictive nature of smoking, smokers' tolerance to nicotine, and the experience of withdrawal symptoms were also examined. Part 2 involved the measurement of physiological and subjective responses in smoking and non-smoking subjects. Electrical changes in the brain, variation in moods, and the purposes of smoking were explored. Part 3 focused on human performance. Smoking behavior patterns were explored by manipulation of the smoking experience (type, strength of cigarette, situation and mood when smoking). The effect of smoking on concentration and cognitive performance and a critical analysis of the experimental procedures used to assess smoking and performance were presented. Part 4 was focussed on attitudes, interventions and social policy. The effects of passive smoking on individual discomfort, health and working efficiency were considered. The relationship between an individual's attitude to smoking, their smoking pattern, and their ability to stop was explored. Interventions included several large-scale prevention and cessation studies in American Schools. Finally the futures of tobacco use and smoking research were considered.

148.   Owen, N., Borland, R., & Hill, D. (1991). Regulatory influences on health-related behaviours: The case of workplace smoking-bans. Australian Psychologist, 26(3), 188-191.

Studies, which showed that workplace bans on smoking result in changes in the behavior and attitudes of smokers, were reviewed. Many public and private organizations in Australia and around the world have recognized the risk of exposure to environmental tobacco smoke to nonsmokers. They have implemented smoking bans in both work places and public places. The main emphasis has been on the effect on the health of the nonsmoker. Smoking bans have also affected the behavior, attitudes and perception of smokers. Most surveys have found approval of smoking bans by nonsmokers and ex-smokers more than smokers. Even smokers often show about 40% approval. Surveys after implementation of the bans often show additional positive support. Changes in smoking behavior often report smoking reductions during work hours. Studies generally showed that compensation after hours for these reductions did not occur. Ethical and social issues about smoking restrictions need careful consideration and were discussed in depth. It was concluded that work place smoking bans benefit both the smoker and the nonsmoker.

149.   Prochaska, J. O., & Goldstein, M. G. (1991). Process of smoking cessation. Implications for clinicians. Clinics in Chest Medicine, 12, 727-735.

The stages-of-change model for changing smoking behavior was suggested as appropriate for most smokers. The 5 stages were: pre-contemplation, contemplation, preparation, action, and maintenance and relapse. They were defined via smokers' attitudes and behavior. Studies which investigated differences between smokers at different stages were reviewed. An intervention selected to match the stage of the particular client was suggested as the best way to promote a change in smoking behavior, for smokers not prepared to quit. The influence of physicians in promoting behavior change was discussed. A stage-matched approach for clinicians was presented. Both assessment of the client's current stage, and appropriate interventions was recommended. It was concluded that the role of the physician, and the use of the stages-of-change model both were important to promote changes in smoking behavior.

150.   Matson, D. M., Lee, J. W., & Hopp, J. W. (1993). The impact of incentives and competitions on participation and quit rates in worksite smoking cessation programs. American Journal of Health Promotion, 7(4), 270-280.

A review was conducted of the incentive and competition-based programs for smoking cessation in worksites. Incentive programs involved cash or prizes paid to participants for quitting smoking. Incentive competitions involved groups that competed for prizes, for having the largest smoking cessation rate. Fifteen quasi-experimental and experimental studies were reviewed. The effects of incentives and competition were distinct from other intervention effects in 8 studies. One study separated effects of competition from incentives. All studies showed positive smoking cessation and reduction outcomes post-intervention. None of the studies reviewed showed that incentives and/or competiton enhanced smoking cessation after 6 months. Five studies however showed enhanced smoking reduction. Three studies showed increased participation rates. It was concluded that work-site incentives/competition intervention programs might be useful to increase participation and smoking reduction. It was suggested that future research is required about long-term effectiveness of incentives, and the types of effective incentives.

151.   Baldwin, S., & Rogers, P. (1996). Controlled smoking (part I): A last resort? Journal of Substance Misuse, 1, 67-73.

Three main issues were addressed about the effects of smoking and smoking modification. Public health policy has influenced smoking modification. Chemicals found in cigarettes, and mortality and morbidity rates due to smoking were reported. Brand-switching interventions and changes in smoker topography were discussed. Smoking psychopharmacology included a description of the addictive nature of nicotine and its biological effect. Nicotine replacement, addiction and withdrawal were also discussed. Controlled smoking was recommended as a last resort for heavy smokers to minimize the desire for tobacco and reduce individual physical harm. The effect of smoking and smoking reduction on heart disease was reported. Psychological factors of smoking, ranging from reports of relaxation to stimulation were discussed. Behavioral assessment for program selection included a discussion using the stages-of-change model. A need was identified for treatment matching for individual smokers according to their individual stage-of-change. Methods of behavioral assessment and appropriate selection of intervention were discussed. It was recommended that controlled smoking should not be overlooked as an appropriate intervention for some smokers.

152.   Baldwin, S. & Rogers, P. (1996). Controlled smoking (part II): A last resort. Journal of Substance Misuse, 1, 142-148.

The need was identified for controlled smoking programs as one important element of public health policy. An historical perspective of smoking identified the use of controlled smoking in the past. The current status of public health policy was described. This consisted of primary prevention programs and cessation programs. The need for controlled smoking as a harm reduction strategy for smokers who did not want to quit (or who are unable to quit) was emphasized. The effects of controlled smoking on passive smoking were also presented. Public health perspectives were presented on smoking, including health promotion aspects and media campaigns. Evaluation factors included political, industrial, and societal interests, with an impact on policy implementation. An explanation and history of controlled smoking was presented. Single-case studies and group studies of controlled smoking research were critically analyzed. Directions for future research were suggested.

153.   Reid, D. (1996). Tobacco control: Overview. Medical British Bulletin, 52, 108-120.

The efficacy, number of smokers influenced, and cost-effectiveness of the principal components of an effective tobacco control programme was assessed. Tobacco control programs included components of public health policy to reduce tobacco advertising, increased taxation to increase cigarette prices, restrictions on smokers for regulation of smoking in public places, and regulation of tar and nicotine content of cigarettes. Interventions and prevention were aimed primarily at youths (including school health education), interpersonal interventions, mass media campaigns, and restrictions on sales. Interventions and cessation aimed at adult smokers included interpersonal advice (both to the general public and from health professionals), and population level intervention (smoking restrictions in public places, paid mass media advertising, and interventions during pregnancy). General interventions were reviewed for all age groups for fiscal policy, health warnings, product modification, bans on cigarette advertising and promotion, and mass communications. It was concluded that many different large-scale efforts all reduced smoking. Health professionals could have a greater impact through the media than through personal advice.

154.   Walker, R. E., & Froggatt, P. (1996). Product modification. British Medical Bulletin, 52, 193-205.

The effects of product modification of low-tar/nicotine cigarettes were investigated. Interest in the 'less harmful' cigarette in the 1950s and 1960s promoted investigation of reconstituted tobacco sheets, filters, and tar reduction. Tobacco substitutes and additives, designed to replace some of the natural tobacco, were reviewed. The potential health 'harm' reduction of lower tar-yields in cigarettes was discussed, with consideration of the effects of smokers' topographical changes and compensatory smoking. Consideration was given to the effects of reduced nicotine yield, carbon monoxide, and other smoke components. The effects of product modification on smoking- related diseases were reviewed. It was concluded that there was evidence to indicate that smoke intake has been reduced. Cigarette modification was described to help reduce the number of premature deaths from tobacco.

7

MISCELLANEOUS

155. Schwarz, N., Servay, W. & Kumpf, M. (1985). Attribution of arousal
      as a mediator of the effectiveness of fear-arousing communications.
      Journal of Applied Social Psychology, 15 (2), 178-188.

Forty-nine male subjects who smoked an average of 15.8 cpd were
recruited from a German university for a study and told that the study
was an evaluation of a new pill in changing galvanic skin response.
Three groups received a placebo pill that was described as having
either an arousing side-effect, tranquillising side-effect, or no side-
effect. Subjects watched a fear-arousing anti-smoking movie and then
had their galvanic skin response assessed. Subjects completed a
questionnaire to assess their attitudes towards smoking. They were told
to monitor their smoking for 2 weeks. A control group completed the
questionaries and self-monitoring but were not exposed to the film and
did not receive the pill.

As expected, all the experimental groups indicated self-reported fear
that was significantly greater the control group. The group who
expected the pill to have a tranquillizing effect reported significantly
greater fear than those expecting no side effects. Subjects expecting
arousing side-effects reported less fear (non-significant). All subjects
who saw the film indicated intentions of greater smoking reduction
than the control group who did not see the film. Subjects expecting a
tranquillizing effect from the placbo pill reported the greatest intentions of smoking reductions , followed by no effect, and then arousing
effect. Subjects who expected no effect from the pill reported a reduction in smoking equivalent to their intentions. They were significantly

different from the control indicating the film had an influence. Subjects who expected a tranquillising effect reported similar reductions to the no effect group. Those subjects who expected an arousing effect reported reductions, but not significantly different from the control group. The implications of these results were discussed in terms of the use of fear arousing communication as a strategy for changing behavior.

8

DISCUSSION

The previous seven chapters highlight the many and varied treatment approaches that have been used to investigate controlled or reduced smoking. This chapter gives an overall picture of the literature on controlled or reduced smoking. The most common methods of data collection, characteristics of smokers, and the methods of treatment for the reduction of smoking are described. The general trend of the treatment's performance in the literature in terms of maintained reductions are discussed. There are many aspects in the research designs frequently found in the controlled or reduced smoking literature that require careful consideration in the design of future research. These included subject selection and assignment, the use of control groups, the goals and hypotheses, attrition and incomplete data, follow-up periods, and method of calculating smoking reductions.

METHOD OF DATA COLLECTION

The most common form of data collection was self-monitoring which used several recording schedules and methods:

1. A card was placed beneath the cellophane wrapper of the cigarette packet and each cigarette was recorded on this card either before or after consumption.
2. A wrist counter was worn and a button pressed after the consumption of each cigarette, and the total recorded after a specific duration.
3. The number of cigarettes smoked was calculated from the packets consumed and recorded on a table or chart at a specific duration.

4. The number of cigarettes smoked was estimated and recorded on a table or chart for a specified duration.
5. The butt of each cigarette was placed in a pouch after consumption, and the pouch was returned to the experimenter after a specified duration. (Number of butts in the pouch was not counted by the subject).
6. The subject bought or was given packets of cigarettes from the experimenter and returned all packets (empty, partially used or full) after a specific duration.
7. The subject delegated a 'significant other' who was contacted by the experimenter to verify the subject's self-report.

Another form of data collection made use of pharmacological methods:

1. Breath carbon monoxide (CO) levels were measured using an 'Ecolyzer CO Analyzer'.
2. Blood nicotine/cotinine, plasma thiocyanate (SCN) and carboxy-haemoglobin (COHb) levels were measured from venous blood samples.
3. Saliva nicotine/cotinine levels were measured using gas chromatography, and saliva thiocyanate levels using spectrophotometric analysis.
4. Consumed cigarette butt length and weight provided an indirect measure of smoking intensity and toxicity; tar and CO exposure increases logarithmically as cigarette length decreases.

CHARACTERISTICS OF SMOKERS

Many studies have been designed to explore the physiological and psychological effects of smoking and differences between groups of smokers.

The physiological effects of low tar/nicotine cigarettes have been investigated. One study reported no significant increase in cigarette consumption from usual to low tar cigarettes (103). Another study reported consumption increased when using low-strength and very low-strength compared to medium-strength cigarettes (97). Carboxyhaemoglobin levels decreased when using low-strength cigarettes and significantly decreased for very-low strength cigarettes compared to medium-strength cigarettes (96, 97). More complete smoking of low and very low strength cigarettes was observed by shorter butt length and analysis of nicotine content of the filter (97). Another study found plasma nicotine and blood COHb levels indicated self-titration of nicotine and CO (119). Mouth level intake of nicotine significantly decreased. Plasma nicotine levels substantially decreased in the comparison of usual and low tar cigarette consumption (103). No significant changes were observed in COHb levels, plasma thiocyanate, puff volume, puff rate, or cigarette duration. This suggested the degree of compensation was only partial (103). A comparison of pregnant and non-pregnant smokers showed no significant differences in puff frequency, consumption changes during brand switching, cigarette duration, nicotine intake or smoking rate. Pregnant smokers were observed to have lower and less variable COHb and SCN levels than non-pregnant smokers (125). These physiological findings suggested that very low tar and nicotine cigarettes decrease the hazards of smoking by reducing the CO and nicotine intake (97, 103).

Smoking has been significantly associated with lung cancer, chronic bronchitis, and ischaemic heart disease in smokers under the age of 55 years (106). Smokers of high-tar cigarettes (29mg+) have twice the risk of chronic bronchitis than smokers of medium-tar cigarettes (17-22mg). Smokers of low-tar cigarettes have a reduced risk of smoking-related illness compared to regular smokers (106). The risk of lung cancer significantly decreased for long-term ex-smokers (106). Smokers of filter cigarettes were not found to have a lower Coronary Heart Disease incidence rate than non-filter smokers, (even after adjustments were made for age, systolic blood pressure, and serum cholesterol (101). A study of patient perception of susceptibility to illness, self-efficacy and changes in smoking behavior found that subjects with high perceived susceptibility and high expectations of efficacy were more likely to reduce smoking after 3 months than subjects of low perceived susceptibility and low expectations of efficacy (124).

Tobacco 'chippers' were defined as regular smokers of 5 or fewer cpd and seem to be unaffected by deprivation. Chippers eliminated nicotine at the same rate as regular smokers and do not maintain a significant plasma nicotine concentration between cigarettes. They may not be motivated to smoke by withdrawal avoidance (109). In a random population-representative survey, 83% of respondents were smokers, of which 8.2% were classified as chippers (113). In this sub-sample chippers did not perceive quitting as difficult, bought smaller packs, had not been given cessation advice from a physician and generally smoked their first cigarette more than 30 minutes after waking. One study described smokers with similar characteristics to chippers as stable very-light smokers who smoked as a social activity with a large emphasis on pleasurable relaxation (112). They were not found to be novice smokers or felt pressure to limit smoking, and they differed from regular smokers in educational level and familial smoking patterns (112). Chippers have been found to inhale and absorb as much nicotine as regular smokers (127). When regular smokers were restricted to the same smoking rate as chippers, regular smokers compensated by extracting more nicotine from each cigarette. This produced an increased blood cotinine concentration compared to chippers (127).

One study of self initiated attempts to reduce cigarette consumption found successful reducers were more motivated to personal change. They used more techniques more frequently, consistently and longer. Successful reducers used positive feedback, self-reinforcement techniques, and problem-solving procedures. These reducers rated their techniques as more practical than unsuccessful reducers (99). Subjects with a high desire to stop, and high internal locus of control, tended to resist relapse (104). Self-efficacy was the only significant Social Cognitive Theory (SCT) predictor for smoking reductions in smokers diagnosed with COPD. Other SCT variables (outcome expectancies and motivational factors) contributed to smoking reduction but not independently from self-efficacy (107). Another study using value and action models found that smoking behavior might be better explained by *desires and emotional states* than *belief and values* (105). The influence of non-specific factors such as motivation, beliefs and expectations, on the reduction of smoking was investigated using Israli kibbutzim subjects. One group was told that they showed strong willpower and the ability to control and change their behavior from analysis of projective tests. This group showed significantly greater reductions post-treatment, and follow-up, than subjects who were told they were randomly selected or control subjects (100).

Studies of pregnant smokers found breath CO to be a valid objective measure of smoking status in pregnancy (102). Maintained reduction during pregnancy was related to age of smoking onset (110). Age, smoking history prior to pregnancy, and partner support were important predictors of successful reductions during pregnancy (102, 108, 110, 114).

The effect of social limitation and influences on smoking behavior has also been investigated. A study of the perceived effect of a tax increase on cigarettes found that smokers expected they would stop or cut down cigarette consumption. The reduction amount was proportional to the size of the tax increase (98). A telephone survey of information about work-site smoking policies found that people employed in non-smoking work-sites were less likely to be current smokers. They were also more likely to never have smoked than employees in smoking work-sites (111). The surveyors also found that people generally reduce smoking on workdays as a result of work-site smoking policies compared to non-work days.

METHOD OF TREATMENT AND GENERAL TRENDS OF RESULTS

Many methods of intervention to stop, reduce or control smoking behavior have been reported, and have been grouped into six main categories.

Self-monitoring, Information, Encouragement and Reinforcement

Self-monitoring is a procedure by which the subject recorded the frequency or rate of self-smoking behavior at specified time periods (e.g. continuous, daily, weekly). Results showed that pre-recording (prior to cigarette consumption) was more effective in creating reductions than post-recording (after cigarette consumption). Continuous recording was the most accurate, demanding, and most effective in promoting changes to smoking behavior (6, 7). Self-monitoring alone did not automatically produce lasting changes in smoking behavior (10, 52, 53). In a comparison of positive (recording successful resistance to smoking urges) and negative (unsuccessful resistance to smoking urges) self-monitoring, it was found that negative self-monitoring was slightly more effective than positive (4).

Non-specific advice and suggestions for smoking reduction showed strong post-treatment effects, modestly maintained at 6 month follow-up in one study (51) and rapid deterioration to baseline in another (55). Significant changes in attitude measures and an increase in motivation to reduce smoking was also found using non-specific advice (122). It was generally found that coping strategies and relapse prevention information improved maintenance of initial reductions (33, 38, 55).

Direct suggestion informed subjects to reduce smoking behavior on their own and also that 'gimmicks' could not help them. Results showed that initial reductions were not well-maintained (43, 46).

Information in the form of direct personal presentation, video and pamphlets showed health risks and methods of reduction/cessation. Results with pregnant smokers showed small reductions and large attrition rates (66, 130).

Physician advice during a medical consultation outlined the implications of smoking and advice on reduction/cessation, again showed small reductions and large attrition rates with pregnant smokers (66). A study of outpatients of a Veterans Administration Medical Clinic found smokers with low levels of behavioral reactance responded better to high amounts of advice. Subjects with high behavioral reactance produced greatest reductions following small amounts of negatively-toned advice (93).

Therapist contact during maintenance often occurred in the form of a phone call or a brief follow-up interview. This showed that despite relapse, smoking was still lower than baseline at 6-months follow-up (46, 54) but not at 12 months (54). Therapist contact during treatment and maintenance in high-contact self-control, rapid-smoking, or normal-paced smoking compared to minimal-contact self-control reported no significant differences. This indicated high-therapist contact may not be warranted (78).

Badge wearing reinforcement involved subjects to wear a badge saying "I don't smoke" to decrease social influences. Results showed that some subjects did not wear the badge and the process was no more effective than self-monitoring alone (52).

Monetary rewards were offered for reductions in cigarette intake measured by afternoon expired air CO levels compared to baseline. The extent of reductions directly related to the amount of reward (26). Changes were made in daytime smoking rather then evening smoking when CO samples were recorded during the day (123). Reductions in CO levels measured during intervention often failed to return to baseline when the monetary rewards were withdrawn (123). Subjects who used a specific plan involving diet changes and activities incompatible with smoking were most successful in achieving reductions (18). Treatment involving self-punishment (donating money to a charity when reduction goals were not met) was more effective than self-reward alone (57).

Token reinforcement was randomly awarded by different staff members to psychiatric outpatients who were not smoking. The tokens (in the form of a lapel button saying "Thank-you for not smoking") were exchanged for merchandize on designated days. Smoking was reduced by over 70% and the intervention was described as easily administered, cost-effective and successful (120).

Drugs or Smoking Alternatives

Buspirone is a nonsedative antianxiety agent used to minimize withdrawal symptoms. Results showed sustained reductions of the urge to smoke and minimization of cravings, withdrawal anxiety, fatigue and weight gain (35).

Fluoxetine is a selective serotonin uptake inhibitor which decreased eating and produces weight loss. Fluoxetine was supplied to subjects who decreased nicotine intake by more than 50%. Weight gain and food intake was significantly reduced in treatment subjects compared to a placebo control (128).

Transdermal nicotine patches filled with a nicotine-based solution were placed on the nondominant forearm of the smoker to provide an alternative 'safer' nicotine source. Cigarette consumption of hospitalized psychiatric patients with the patches was substantially decreased. Urine nicotine output also decreased, which demonstrated its effectiveness to reduce cigarette consumption (126).

Placebo pill was used to investigate the symptom or efficacy attribution corresponding to smoking reductions and withdrawal effects. The pill was described to either increase symptoms, decrease symptoms or the effect on symptoms was not mentioned (symptoms attribution). After reductions, subjects were told that 50% of their reductions were achieved by their own effort (efficacy attribution). Results showed increased self-efficacy produced greater reductions than drug efficacy (13).

Refined cigarette smoke was the production of a smoke condensate from a machine-smoked cigarette that can be placed in a cigarette-sized tube and heated to allow the smoker to inhale vapours. This provided the familiar sensory cues of smoking while greatly reducing intake of nicotine. Many harmful gases normally found in cigarette smoke were absent. Subjective and biochemical results suggested that to reduce harm, refined smoke is a viable alternative to smoking (32).

Smokeless tobacco (as an alternative nicotine source to cigarette smoking) has been found to decrease annual deaths from smoking and related health costs by reducing health risk. Even after long and heavy tobacco smoking history, the transition to smokeless tobacco has been achieved and well-maintained (42).

Hypnosis

Hypnosis is the presentation of anti-smoking or smoking reduction messages to subjects in a trance-like state often induced by progressive deep muscle relaxation. Messages are presented to subjects in a variety of forms including:

1. direct suggestion, positive reinforcement and motivational instructions for stopping
2. role-playing where the subject acts the role of the non-smoker
3. desensitization which pairs the relaxing effects of hypnosis with the physiological withdrawal effects of not smoking
4. stimulus control in which subjects reduce the places and times of smoking.

Most studies fail to find significant correlations between smoking reductions and hypnotizability among treated subjects. Most subjects report the therapeutic role of hypnosis as minimal. Abstinence which is maintained for 3-4 months has been found to contain a high probability of long-term success (14, 20, 37). Results from hypnotic treatment compared to the same treatment without the hypnotic inductions showed no difference in reductions, which returned to baseline by 3 months follow-up (68). Hypnosis to reduce smoking in a deaf patient made use of induction through lip reading. The procedure successfully reduced smoking from 60 cpd to an average of 2 cpd maintained during a 9-month follow-up (116).

Stimulus Control

Work-site smoking restrictions placed limitations of availability of time and places available for smoking in the workplace. Analysis of a hospital-wide smoking ban showed that smoking reductions during work hours were generally not compensated via increased smoking outside of work. Pharmacological analysis suggests smoking ban intervention provided a limited health benefit for tobacco exposure reduction with only minor withdrawal discomfort (39). A random telephone survey found that reduction in smoking on work days compared to non-work days was a result of worksite smoking policies (111).

Relaxation of specific craving spots on the human body or of non-specific areas during imagined scenes produced no significant smoking reductions post-treatment in one study (47) but significant reductions in others (9, 48) with slight relapse. Relaxation in place of smoking during an imagined situation that led to the desire to smoke was administered by phone to subjects at their home every 1.5 hours for a 24-hour period. Initial reductions of 40% of baseline had relapsed by a 12-month follow-up (115).

Cue exposure involved identification of smoking situation or cues and devising alternative actions for each situation. Results showed moderate success in maintaining smoking reductions (36, 55) but relapse by 12 months follow-up (55).

Self-regulation therapy associated a word or cue with a sensation from a physical stimulus so the sensation can be reproduced without the physical stimulus. Results showed initial success with self-controlled smokers, abstainers and reducers, but treatment outcomes were best maintained by self-controlled smokers (40).

Covert sensitization paired an undesirable act with an aversive consequence to elicit reductions in desirability of the target behavior. Most reductions were inferior to rapid smoking (76), and had returned to baseline by 2-month and 4-month follow-up (15, 23, 47). Some studies found that although relapse had occurred, follow-up reductions were still significantly less than baseline (46). One study suggested that attention or suggestion was a valid interpretation for the effectiveness of covert sensitization (43).

Covert modeling involved imagined scenes which included an urge to smoke but making an alternative non-smoking response and receiving favorable consequences for not smoking. Results showed this procedure was no more effective than self-monitoring. Reductions could be explained by non-specific factors (10).

Thought stopping involved the visualization of a situation in which an urge to smoke was experienced, followed by a loud handclap and a voice yelled 'stop'. Progressively, the voice whispered 'stop' and finally subvocalizing it. Subjects were encouraged to practice this procedure in real situations. Results showed modest maintenance of large reductions (47, 52).

Habit reversal involved understanding motivation, awareness training, competing response training and public display procedures. Results showed rapid and impressive abstinence/reduction rates with moderate relapse (51). A similar procedure called Eliminating Self-Defeating Behaviors reported significant reductions in daily smoking, maintained at 4 weeks follow up (79).

Systematic Desensitization

Situational typing involves the successive gradual reduction in smoking in low-risk, medium-risk and high-risk situations. Results showed significant reductions with varying but generally slight relapse (38, 43).

Controlled smoking involved brand switching to achieve a 50% reduction of nicotine content, 50% reduction of percentage of each cigarette smoked and 50% reduction in number of cigarettes smoked. Individual goal-setting and information on relapse prevention was often included. Results show subjects often achieved goal reductions in nicotine content but only 25% reductions in percentage of each cigarette smoked and number of cigarettes smoked. All reductions were well maintained at 6-month follow-up suggesting reliable and moderately successful long-term results (22, 60, 61). Partner support aided maintenance efforts. *Gradual* reductions were better at producing long-term effects than *abrupt* reductions (25, 60, 61). One study presented subjects in a cessation program that failed with a controlled smoking alternative. The non-abstainers presented with the controlled smoking alternative did not show greater reductions than non-abstainers not presented with the controlled smoking alternative (65).

Graduated filters can be fitted to a cigarette to induce reductions in nicotine, tar, carbon monoxide, and other poisonous gases when smoking. Results showed that the filter system successfully reduced tobacco exposure, without signs of compensation indicating reduced health risk (16).

Smoking chair restricted smoking to all situations (other than sitting in a specific chair) in the absence of social situations or items of interest (e.g. television or books). Control of smoking to a predetermined rate, and eventually cessation was achieved and maintained using this method of smoking in the absence of environmental stimuli (1).

Brand fading involved progressive brand changes to cigarettes containing lower nicotine/tar/carbon monoxide levels. Although one study found the health benefit of smoking a 'safer' brand at the same rate to be questionable (24), interpretation of most studies found that brand fading produced successful reduction/cessation results (17, 21, 45, 53, 56, 89). The addition of anxiety management did not produce the desired effects with high-anxiety smokers (86). Self-instruction and self-efficacy training did not increase treatment effectiveness for reduction, but self-efficacy training aided cessation (89).

Smoking reductions in rate, followed by maintenance strategies in a non-aversive behavioral approach produced impressive reductions. These reductions were maintained by more than half the sample at 3 and 4-year follow-up (19). Another study showed that therapist-paced goal setting showed greater maintenance of reductions at 3-month follow-up than subject-paced reductions (58).

Increasing delay training increased the delay between puffs by 10 seconds on every trial and interpretation of results indicated the procedure produces superior self-control than rapid smoking on an 'urge temptation task' (59).

Punishment and Aversive Conditioning

Hot, smoky air was blown into the face of the smoker whilst the subject smoked, and fresh air was substituted when the subject extinguished the cigarette. Results showed than initial reductions were poorly maintained at follow-up (3, 44).

Rapid smoking consisted of inhaling a cigarette on command every 6 seconds until it could no longer be tolerated. Often the procedure was repeated after a short rest period. Results showed impressive reductions from baseline with only average maintenance (8, 44). Rapid smoking was superior in both reductions and abstinence rates compared to covert sensitization and its combination (76). Rapid smoking combined with controlled smoking procedures improved abstinence results. Rapid smoking also aided smokers who did not wish to quit completely (77). Abstinence and reduction rates were not enhanced by self-control, relaxation or contingency contracts. One study found the procedure no more effective then simple support (55). Another study found it achieved equivalent reductions to increasing delay training but lower resistance to temptation (59).

Satiation increased consumption of cigarettes (doubled or tripled) for a time period to diminish the reinforcement value and to reduce smoking behavior. Results showed gradual reductions with varying maintenance (2, 48).

Shock involved the punishment of actual smoking behavior by administration of a 'barely tolerable' electric shock delivered contingently, based on actual smoking behaviors (inhaling, exhaling, etc.). This treatment was followed by electric shock punishment to imagined smoking situations. Results showed that neither placebo shock, therapist-delivered shock, nor subject-delivered shock maintained reductions at follow-up (50). The use of shock for the reduction of smoking was not supported.

Sensory deprivation was conducted in a shielded, dark, sound-reducing chamber containing a hospital bed, chemical toilet and water and vanilla-flavored diet food available via tubes when lying on the bed. Subjects were dressed in simple garments and told to lie still for the duration of treatment (usually a 24-hour period). Results showed good reductions and maintenance at 12-month follow-up (90, 115). No difference was found between addicted and pre-addicted smokers (level of psychological commitment to smoking) after sensory deprivation intervention (115).

CONSIDERATIONS AND LIMITATIONS

Overall, the large volume of research assessing the effectiveness of different strategies to achieve controlled or reduced smoking indicate several methods that give modest outcomes, and many methods that give poor outcomes. However, before drawing firm conclusions from these results, the limitations of the research should be considered.

Subject Selection

The studies presented a wide range of subject recruitment methods and selection for treatment and intervention. Due to the specific characteristics of the samples of smokers used in many studies, generalizing results to the average smoker, or particularly to the heavy smoker (most likely to be in need of intervention) is very difficult.

Some studies used a university student population, with associated problems of generalization to the normal population. The average university smoker was young (18-24). Typically students have a briefer, lighter smoking history. Also, often students may not have a strong desire to quit or reduce smoking. Many students have participated in experiments to meet their academic study requirements or for extra credit. The same treatment performed given to a student sample and to a sample of mature heavy smokers (who have expressed a strong desire to reduce smoking) will produce different outcomes.

Most studies have recruited subjects through newspaper, radio or television advertisements. People who responded to these advertisements often have been enthusiastic about the treatment. Subjects have been motivated to achieve the desired goal, and to fulfil the requirements of the study. This has enabled experimenters to target specific groups of people of different age, gender, health, educational level, and socioeconomic status through the area of circulation and type of media used in advertisement.

Some studies have recruited subjects using a physician referral. This method has been used particularly in studies focussed on populations with health conditions (pregnancy, and factors associated with or diagnosis of smoking-related disease/illness).

Subject Assignment

The random assignment of subjects into treatment and control groups has not always been reported, which has created problems of bias. Many experiments have matched treatment and control groups on variables such as number, gender, age, baseline number of years smoking, and baseline smoking rate. Attrition and incomplete data collection at follow-up sometimes has produced unmatched groups. This was especially relevant when a particular kind of smoker (e.g. heavy or very addicted smokers) were not represented in a group to which they were originally assigned. For example, subjects who responded to an advertisement with a strong desire to quit (or reduce) smoking but were placed in a control group with treatment delay. Such subjects may have lost interest and not provided accurate information or started self-help or external smoking intervention. The dynamics of the control group in this example would have changed and were not equivalent to the pre-treatment attitudes and behavior of subjects. Health reasons may have prevented some subjects from receiving a particular treatment. This was particularly true in studies that involved rapid smoking as a treatment. In all studies, subjects who became pregnant (and subjects with cardiovascular or chronic respiratory problems) were excluded from rapid smoking treatment. Such subjects may have been assigned to a different treatment group, which could affect the group response to treatment.

Control Groups

Control groups were often matched to treatment groups with variables such as number, age, gender, mean baseline smoking rate and number of years smoking. Attrition of control group subjects has sometimes created unmatched groups. This has resulted in inaccurate comparisons and exaggerated treatment effects. Debate about the therapeutic effects of the self-monitoring of smoking behavior has created data collection problems. This was especially true in obtaining correct and accurate smoking behavior data from a control group. Collection of data may have affected the results. Continuous self-monitoring was the most accurate method to obtain smoking data. Continuous self-monitoring has also been found to produce a small treatment effect. Estimated smoking rates at weekly intervals has been found to have no treatment effects. It is however an inaccurate method. Some studies have lacked a control group, or have failed to produce follow-up data for control groups for comparison with treatment groups. The absence of a control group creates the possibility that some other event that coincided with the experimental manipulation was responsible for the outcome.

Treatment or Study Goals/Hypotheses

Two main groups of studies were formed in this category. The first group had a goal of producing controlled or reduced smoking. The second group had an abstinence goal. Reports of reductions in studies with a goal of abstinence should be given careful consideration. The subject may have felt that a slight relapse after a cessation period (or even not achieving abstinence) was a failure according to the goals of the study. Relapse near to baseline has sometimes occurred. A study with a goal of 'maintained reduction' would have given these subjects achievable goals, despite the temporary setback of a relapse. The goals of the study should be made clear to the subjects at the recruitment stage. Interventions should be appropriate to meet the needs and desires of the smoker.

Attrition and Incomplete Data

In any study subjects can drop out unexpectedly which can cause uneven group size and produce incomplete data sets. The occurrence of incomplete data at follow-up assessments (especially if extended periods of time were involved) was common, as not all subjects could be contacted. In the studies reported here the most common reason for subjects to withdraw from the study was pregnancy, or after physician advice. Most studies counted drop-outs as treatment failures. Some studies excluded all data, including baseline and initial treatment data of subjects who did not complete treatment. Other studies included the baseline and initial treatment data and simply adjusted the number of subjects for any data manipulations.

Follow-up Periods

The general trend reported by McFall & Hamen (4) suggested a V-shaped curve can often describe the treatment effects of smoking studies. A large initial decrease from baseline smoking rate during and at the end of treatment (often about 30-40% of baseline), is followed by a gradual asymptotic relapse to near 75% of baseline levels at follow-ups. Complete relapse to baseline has been reported, but smoking rates rarely exceed baseline measures at follow-up. The number and time period post-treatment of the follow-up data collection points are crucial to a well-planned and executed study. The studies which do include follow-up data, often do not extend follow-ups past 3 months (and those that do rarely extend past 12 months). Studies with data reported for only short follow-up periods need to be considered carefully as often apparently successful and impressive reduction rates with little relapse may be a result of subjects at the bottom of the curve. Studies which have *short* follow-up periods provide useful information of initial success and show where further research is needed. Studies which have *long* follow-up periods give a better indication of treatment validity.

Another tendency reported by McFall & Hamen (4) is the 'floor effect' where subjects reduce smoking to 10 or fewer cigarettes per day but do not achieve abstinence. The floor effect was noted with non-abstainers in another study, but was not maintained at a 12 month follow-up (88). This phenomenon of 'stuck points' was also reported at 10-12 cpd by Hills (58). Stuck points at 24.6, 13.1 and 12.0cpd were reported by Levinson, Shapiro, Schwartz & Tursky with most subjects not achieving sustained reductions below 12.0cpd (70). The replicated occurrence of the floor effect in the literature lends support to the area of controlled smoking. It highlights the need to incorporate reduction goals in cessation intervention designs to ensure the needs of all smokers (including those who can not or do not want to quit) are met.

Elevated Reduction Levels by Including Abstainers

Many studies report a group's overall reduction rate post-treatment and at follow-up periods. Following treatment however, most groups can be divided into abstainer and non-abstainers. The overall reduction level from baseline becomes inflated in a group which includes abstainers, which gives the potential for misleading results and conclusions. Following treatment, all studies should further divide each group into abstainers and non-abstainers, and perhaps further divide non-abstainers into reducers (or controlled smokers) and relapsers (those who relapse to baseline at follow up). This will ensure that accurate conclusions are drawn from cessation, reduction and relapse rates.

Overall, it becomes clear through careful analysis that the literature on controlled or reduced smoking is plagued with methodological flaws. In addition, the majority of the literature on controlled or reduced smoking appears to have the aims and objectives of smoking cessation research. There is clear evidence in the literature that there is a population of smokers who are regular, but very light smokers. There is also evidence from several authors that smokers attempting to reduce or quit smoking reach "stuck points" before cessation, and can maintain regular, light smoking without relapse. A large number of studies investigating a broad array of different treatments have been presented. Overall, considering outcome and methodology, few treatments have produced the results required to facilitate major development of reduced or controlled smoking programs to cater for the needs of smokers who cannot or do not want to quit smoking completely. Well planned and executed research is required to extend the research in controlled or reduced smoking to advance the services for smokers who wish to achieve sustained reductions.

CONCLUSION

The already-published literature from the 1960s through the 1990s has confirmed the impression of a biomedical conceptual orthodoxy, in both treatment and prevention services. Specifically, smoking has been viewed within a structural framework which presented the index behavior as an all-or-nothing phenomenon. Smokers have been characterized in a similar style to people who misuse other addictive substances. The prevailing biomedical orthodoxy in the fields of smoking research and social policy has generated a series of powerful propositions:

1. Smoking is an addiction,
2. Smokers have similar characteristics to people who misuse or abuse other addictive agents (e.g. alcohol, heroin or prescribed drugs) typified by dependence, lack of self-control, helplessness, hopelessness and a personal vulnerability to the substance,
3. Interventions should be focused on physiological aspects of smoking (e.g. withdrawal, craving, physical 'dependence') rather than on psychological aspects of health and lifestyle (e.g. fitness, nutrition, coping, self-esteem),
4. Smoking is an all-or-nothing phenomenon, which creates three sub-populations of non-smokers, smokers and ex-smokers (abstainers who have successfully quit smoking completely),
5. Intervention efforts should be targeted toward 'quit programs' for existing smokers and primary prevention programs for teenage and young adult non-smokers.

This false bifurcation of the field into three groups of smokers/never smoked/ex-smokers has produced several unfortunate consequences.

First, health promotion and prevention resources have been incorrectly directed toward ineffective or weak strategies and programs. Examples included much media/public broadcasting and many school programs, neither of which has produced substantive demonstrable benefits (except financial gains to contracted agencies and organizations).

Second, the sub-population of chronic smokers (who refuse to quit) frequently have been ignored by health educators. Often chronic smokers were not included in a treatment sample, implying that they are 'untreatable'. Where chronic smokers have been included in treatment strategies they have been given puny programs, with unproven outcomes. Chronic smokers have been given the same treatment as less-severe smokers. They also have been expected to achieve the same goal of abstinence. Some ineffective cessation programs have sensitized smokers to subsequent treatment attempts.

Third, the dominant conceptual model of smoking cessation ('stages of change') is deeply flawed. Many would-be non-smokers who seek to quit are poorly served by this model, *which does not include reduced smoking as a sub-goal toward eventual cessation.* 'Stages of change' will shortly be superceded by a new dominant conceptual paradigm.

The failure to correctly identify reduced/attenuated smoking as a 'staging post' to eventual cessation means that incorrect goals frequently have been allocated to smokers. Typically, clinicians and health educators have recommended single-target goals to smokers (i.e. 'total abstinence'). Moreover, with few exceptions, treatments have been focused on an all-or-none approach to smoking cessation. Some quit programs have featured the tapering of cigarette smoking, toward a cessation goal. (The contemporary use of nicotine patches to *fade out* smoking is a relatively recent development). Regardless of individual smoker characteristics, most interventions have been based on relatively unsophisticated cessation goals. Although success was often reported in terms of 'reduction', smokers were rarely given a treatment goal of reduction as an alternative to cessation. Worldwide, thousands of smokers have been sensitized into 'failure scenarios' after implementation of inappropriate treatments. These smokers have been given a strict goal requiring complete abstinence, where a relapse of any kind has been considered treatment failure. The conceptualization of smoking as an all-or-nothing phenomenon has infiltrated public's opinion about smoking. Many smokers believe that if they smoke one cigarette, they may as well smoke more. The education of smokers who do not wish to quit about the benefits of controlled or reduced smoking, will help to diminish the impact of 'failure scenarios'. In addition, implementation of effective treatment strategies with realistic treatment goals will help to establish 'success scenarios'. Smoker competencies will be increased as well as expectations for success and a range of refusal/coping skills.

Treatments focussing on an all-or-nothing approach to smoking cessation generally have had poor outcomes (Baldwin & Rogers, 1996a). Moreover, the existence of a large residual population of treatment-resistant chronic smokers is proof positive of the inadequacy of traditional approaches to smoking reduction and prevention. Typically, contemporary treatment programs have been aimed at smokers in 'action' or in 'contemplation' (Prochaska & Goldstein, 1991). Relapsed smokers frequently have been overlooked in reduction or cessation programs. Too often, chronic smokers have been viewed as 'untreatable'. As a result, of the consequent outgrouping and stereotyping, few resources have been allocated. Most recently, and with spectacular consequences, chronic smokers in the UK have been denied access to national health service resources (eg cardiac surgery) as a result of a *perceived unwillingness to quit smoking*.

Put simply, chronic smokers may require a completely different treatment approach, based on a total reconceptualization of smoking reduction/cessation. This will require acceptance in the smoking research field that the dominant treatment paradigm is faulty. Many chronic smokers have experienced repeated failures from multiple unsuccessful quit attempts. Some smokers have accumulated a personal history of 300-400 unsuccessful quit attempts. In this context, it may be clinically inappropriate and counterproductive to set abstinence as a treatment goal.

Abstinence, although desirable as an end state, in the short-term may be completely unachievable by chronic smokers. Rather, such smokers should aim for *self-control as the primary treatment goal*. The achievement of smoking control may then act as a 'staging post' prior to subsequent abstinence.

It is difficult for many health educators to recommend any goal except abstinence. Especially for clinicians (eg psychologists, medical personnel) and nurses, recommendation of a treatment goal which apparently endorses smoking behavior is anathema. Many health educators have been taught and trained to view abstinence as the sole treatment goal for a range of addictive substances, including alcohol, heroin and 'soft drugs' (eg marijuana). The twin concepts of 'zero tolerance' and 'just say no' policies are both located conceptually within an abstinence framework for substance misuse. Ironically, the empirical evidence is poor, both for zero tolerance and for refusal strategies (Baldwin & Rogers, 1996b).

The promotion of abstinence as a treatment goal has been ideologically driven, not data-driven. Especially in the USA, abstinence approaches have been promoted in the absence of supporting data. Instead, powerful political forces and specific lobby groups have promoted abstinence as the primary treatment goal. In the contemporary cultural climate of 'evidence-based' perspectives in health and medicine, this ideological imperative is a striking contradiction. Rather, there is substantial evidence to support the adoption of a range of treatment approaches. A multi-intervention approach is instead required. Controlled or attenuated smoking should be seen as a legitimate treatment goal for smokers, *en route to subsequent abstinence.*

The acceptance of controlled/attenuated smoking as a legitimate treatment goal produces significant additional clinical consequences. Specifically, for smokers who refuse to quit completely, achievement of a reduced smoking goal may be an acceptable medium-term treatment alternative. The health damage from smoking is dose-dependent (Baldwin & Rogers, 1996a). Smoking fewer cigarettes (instead of many cigarettes) therefore may be an acceptable and viable treatment goal for some clinicians.

Moreover this approach is consistent with the contemporary public health focus on whole-population solutions to health problems. There is a treatment nexus at the intersection between individual behavior change and epidemiological approaches to harm reduction (Winett, Altman & Barthes, 1994). The challenge for health educators working in the area of smoking control will be to correctly identify an appropriate treatment goal for *each individual smoker.* The challenge for researchers in the area of smoking will be to identify the sub-population of chronic smokers (who refuse to quit) that are currently being neglected. Treatment goals and strategies should be established to provide the most *realistic* harm reduction for these smokers.

Hence there is considerable merit in reinvestigation of controlled smoking interventions. There is substantial empirical support for a revised conceptual model, whereby *reduced/controlled/attenuated smoking is viewed as a precursor to eventual cessation.* Equally, for chronic smokers who refuse to quit completely, controlled smoking may be the only treatment that enables harm reduction, and therefore might be considered an appropriate 'treatment of choice'.

REFERENCES

Baldwin, S. & Rogers, P. (1996a). Controlled smoking (part I): A last resort? Journal of Substance Misuse, 1, 67-73.

Baldwin, S. & Rogers, P. (1996b). Controlled smoking (part II): A last resort? Journal of Substance Misuse, 1, 142-148.

Prochaska, J. O., & Goldstein, M. G. (1991). Process of smoking cessation. Implications for clinicians. Clinics in Chest Medicine, 12, 727-735.

Winett, R., Altman, R. A., & Barthes, C. D. (1994). Public Health and Health Psychology: An integrative approach. New York: Allyn & Bacon.

AUTHOR INDEX

SUBJECT INDEX

low activity, 122
low cost, 83, 92, 130
low nicotine, 24, 32, 45, 97, 119,
129, 141, *p114, p115*
low tar level, 17, 24, 32, 96, 97,
129, 140, 141, *p114, p115*
lung cancer, 42, 106, 138, 139,
140, *p115*
lung function, 101, 107
lungs, 12, 139

maintenance stage, 94, 104, 149
manual, 25, 27, 30, 69, 78, 92
material (printed), 71, 77, 94, 143
media, 92, 141, 152, 153, *p124,
p130*
meditative states, 143
messages, 46, 68, 116, 143, *p119*
methodological problems, 8, 135,
136, *p127*
methodological techniques, 135,
p127
minimal contact, 27, 78, 87, 124,
p118
minimal exposure, 145
minimal intervention, 128
modeling, 10, 83, 85, *p120*
models, 21, 36, 83, 85, 105, 122,
132, 149, 151, *p116, p130, p132*
monetary penalty (to charity), 31,
57, 75, *p118*
monetary rewards, 18, 26, 31, 57,
123, 150, *p118*
mood, 38, 39, 40, 63, 105, 147
morbidity rates, 121, 151
mortality, 121, 140, 141, 143, 151
motivation, 4, 10, 26, 42, 51, 88,
91, 99, 100, 107, 112, 122, 133,
137, 145, *p116, p117, p119,
p121*
mouthwashes, 143
multifaceted interventive program,
82

multiple-component treatment, 77,
80, 132, 136, 143
Multiple Risk Factor Intervention
Trial, 121
muscle relaxation training, 23, 46,
91, 118, *p119*
myocardial infarction, 138, 140

nausea, 15, 46
negative advice, 93, *p117*
negative attitude, 108
negative consequences, 48, 73, 105
negative images, 143
negative interactions, 30
negative practice, 5, 74
negative reinforcement, 48
negative self-monitoring, 4, 11,
p117
nicotine addiction/dependence,
113, 143, 151, *p129*
nicotine elimination, 109
nicotine exposure, 29, 127
nicotine fading/reduction, 12, 17,
21, 22, 24, 25, 29, 30, 32, 45,
53, 56, 60, 61, 62, 63, 86, 89,
96, 97, 103, 119, 125, 128, 129,
140, 141, 143, 154, *p119, p121,
p122*
nicotine gum, 42, 136, 143, 146
nicotine patches, 42, 64, 126,
p118, p130
nicotine, role of, 134, 147
nicotine replacement, 143, 151
nicotine tolerance, 109, 147
no contact, 46, 47, 80
no specific instruction, 122
noise, 136
non-aversive, 19, 21, 23, 31, 44,
50, 54, 85, *p122*
non-contingent punishment, 3, 5
non-dependent smokers, 109, 127
non-specific factors, 4, 46, 55, 74,
77, 100, 136, *p116, p120*

About the Compilers

PAMELA ROGERS is a post-graduate student at the University of Western Sydney in Australia.

STEVE BALDWIN is a Professor of Psychology, University of Teesside, School of Social Sciences, Middlesbrough UK. He is the co-author, with Melissa Oxlad, of *Electroshock and Minors* (Greenwood Press, forthcoming).